CLINICAL COMPANION FOR

FUNDAMENTALS
of NURSING:

ACTIVE LEARNING FOR COLLABORATIVE PRACTICE

Barbara L. Yoost, MSN, RN, CNS, CNE, ANEF
Assistant Professor
Division of Nursing
Notre Dame College

Lynne R. Crawford, MSN, RN, MBA, CNE
Retired Faculty
College of Nursing
Kent State University

Subject Matter Expert

Veronica "Ronnie" Peterson, BA RN, BSN, MS
Manager of Clinical Support
University of Wisconsin Medical Foundation
Adjunct Clinical Instructor
University of Wisconsin School of Nursing
Madison, Wisconsin

ELSEVIER

ELSEVIER

3251 Riverport Lane
Maryland Heights, MO 63046

Clinical Companion for Fundamentals of Nursing:
Active Learning for Collaborative Practice   978-0-323-37133-9

Notices

International Standard Book Number: 978-0-323-37133-9

Executive Content Strategist: Tamara Myers
Content Development Manager: Jean Sims Fornango
Publishing Services Manager: Jeff Patterson
Senior Project Manager: Mary Stueck
Design Direction: Julia Dummitt

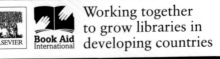

Working together
to grow libraries in
developing countries

www.elsevier.com • www.bookaid.org

Printed in the United States of America

Last digit is the print number: 6 5 4 3 2

Preface

Clinical Companion for Fundamentals of Nursing is designed to be a portable, quick reference for information focused on adult health care. Veronica "Ronnie" Peterson developed this format to help students master the necessary facts and figures needed to practice nursing in today's fast-paced environment. Her students have made it clear that they appreciate the assistance.

"As a nursing student, I value resources of helpful information and practice tips to further my pursuit of a career in nursing. This handy guide is a great asset, with material that is easy to read and comprehend. I will continue to use this book throughout nursing school and in my nursing career.

Ronnie Peterson's years of experience as a nurse and educator helps her provide useful advice for nursing students like me."

Tyler Blaskowski
Viterbo University
La Crosse, Wisconsin

Contents

Preface, iii

Nursing Basics

For more in-depth information on nursing basics, consult the following:

Centers for Disease Control and Prevention: CDC works for you 24-7, 2014. Retrieved from *www.cdc.gov/24-7/*.

The Joint Commission: National patient safety goals, 2014. Retrieved from *www.jointcommission.org/standards_information/npsgs.aspx*.

Yoost BL, Crawford LR: *Fundamentals of nursing: Active learning for collaborative practice*, St. Louis, 2016, Mosby.

CHAPTER 1

Nursing and Professional Practice

ANA CODE OF ETHICS[1]

1. The nurse, in all professional relationships, practices with compassion and respect for the inherent dignity, worth, and uniqueness of every individual, unrestricted by considerations of social or economic status, personal attributes, or the nature of health problems.
2. The nurse's primary commitment is to the patient, whether an individual, family, group, or community.

---

[1]Reprinted with permission from American Nurses Association: *Code of ethics for nurses*, Washington, D.C., 2001, Author.

3. The nurse promotes, advocates for, and strives to protect the health, safety, and rights of the patient.
4. The nurse is responsible and accountable for individual nursing practice and determines the appropriate delegation of tasks consistent with the nurse's obligation to provide optimum patient care.
5. The nurse owes the same duties to self as to others, including the responsibility to preserve integrity and safety, to maintain competence, and to continue personal and professional growth.
6. The nurse participates in establishing, maintaining, and improving health care environments and conditions of employment conducive to the provision of quality health care and consistent with the values of the profession through individual and collective action.
7. The nurse participates in the advancement of the profession through contributions to practice, education, administration, and knowledge development.
8. The nurse collaborates with other health professionals and the public in promoting community, national, and international efforts to meet health needs.
9. The profession of nursing, as represented by associations and their members, is responsible for articulating nursing values, for maintaining the integrity of the profession and its practice, and for shaping social policy.

MASLOW'S HIERARCHY OF NEEDS

Self-Actualization: recognition and realization of one's potential, growth, health, and autonomy

Self-Esteem: self-worth, self-respect, independence, privacy, status, dignity, and self-reliance

Love and Belonging: affection, intimacy, support, and reassurance

Safety and Security: from a physiologic and psychological threat; and protection, stability, and lack of danger

Physiologic Needs: oxygen, food, elimination, temperature control, sex, movement, rest, and comfort

THE HEALTH BELIEF MODEL

Concept	Definition	Potential Change Strategies
Perceived Susceptibility	Beliefs about the chances of getting a condition or disease	Define the populations at risk Tailor risk information based on an individual's characteristics or behaviors

Concept	Definition	Potential Change Strategies
Perceived Susceptibility —cont'd		Help the individual develop an accurate perception of his or her own risk
Perceived Severity	Beliefs about the seriousness of a condition and its consequences	Specify the consequences of a condition and recommend action or intervention
Perceived Benefits	Beliefs about the effectiveness of taking action to reduce risk or seriousness	Explain how, where, and when to take action and what the potential positive results will be
Perceived Barriers	Beliefs about the material and psychological costs of taking action	Offer reassurance, incentives, and assistance; correct misinformation or allegations
Cues to Action	Factors that activate "readiness to change"	Provide "how to" information, promote awareness, and employ reminder systems

Continued

THE HEALTH BELIEF MODEL—cont'd

Concept	Definition	Potential Change Strategies
Self-Efficacy	Confidence in one's ability to take action	Provide training and guidance in performing action Use progressive goal setting Give verbal reinforcement Demonstrate desired behaviors

From National Cancer Institute and U.S. Department of Health and Human Services: *Theory at a glance: A guide for health promotion practices*, ed 2. National Institutes of Health, U.S. Department of Health and Human Services, 2005.

NURSING SPECIALTIES[2]

AD   associate degree nurse

A/NP   adult/nurse practitioner

BS (BSN)   Bachelor of Science (Bachelor of Science in nursing)

CCRN   critical care registered nurse

CDE   certified diabetes educator

CEN   certified emergency nurse

CNE   certified nurse educator

CNM   certified nurse-midwife; clinical nurse manager

CNS   clinical nurse specialist

CRNA   certified registered nurse anesthetist

DN   doctorate in nursing

EdD   doctorate of education

---

[2]From Peterson V: *Clinical companion for fundamentals of nursing: Just the facts*, ed. 8, St. Louis, 2012, Mosby.

FP-NP   family practice nurse practitioner
G-NP   geriatric nurse practitioner
LPN   licensed practical nurse
LVN   licensed vocational nurse
MEd   master of education
MPH   master of public health
MS (MSN)   master of science (master of science in
   nursing)
MSNR   master of science in nursing with research
NP   nurse practitioner
NP/C   nurse practitioner/certified
ONS   oncology nurse specialist
PhD   doctor of philosophy
PhDc   doctor of philosophy, candidate
P-NP   pediatric nurse practitioner
RN   registered nurse
RNA   registered nurse anesthetist
RNC   registered nurse certified
TNCC   trauma nurse core course

NURSING ORGANIZATIONS[3]

AAACN   American Academy of Ambulatory Care
   Nursing
AACCN   American Association of Critical Care
   Nurses
AACN   American Association of Colleges of
   Nursing
AAHN   American Association for the History of
   Nursing, Inc.
AALNC   American Association of Legal Nurse
   Consultants
AAMN   American Assembly for Men in Nursing
AANA   American Association of Nurse Anesthetists;
   American Association of Nurse Attorneys

[3]From Peterson V: *Clinical companion for fundamentals of nursing:
Just the facts,* ed. 8, St. Louis, 2012, Mosby.

AANN   American Association of Neuroscience Nurses

AANP   American Academy of Nurse Practitioners

AAOH   American Association of Occupational Health Nurses, Inc.

AAON   American Association of Office Nurses

AASPIN   American Association of Spinal Cord Injury Nurses

ABNF   Association of Black Nursing Faculty, Inc.

ACCH   Association for the Care of Children's Health

ACHNE   Association of Community Health Nursing Educators

ACHSA   American Correctional Health Services Association

ACNM   American College of Nurse Midwives

ACPN   Advocates for Child Psychiatric Nursing

ACS   American Cancer Society

AHA   American Heart Association

AHNA   American Holistic Nurses Association

ANA   American Nurses Association

ANAC   Association of Nurses in AIDS Care

ANC   Army Nurses Corps

ANF   American Nurses Foundation

ANNA   American Nephrology Nurses' Association

AONE   American Organization of Nurse Executives

AORN   Association of Operating Room Nurses

APHA   American Public Health Association

APIC   Association for Practitioners in Infection Control

APON   Association of Pediatric Oncology Nurses

ARC   American Red Cross

ARN   Association of Rehabilitation Nurses

ASORN   American Society of Ophthalmic Registered Nurses, Inc.

ASPAN   American Society of Post Anesthesia Nurses

ASPRSN   American Society of Plastic and Reconstructive Surgical Nurses, Inc.

ATDNF   Alpha Tau Delta National Fraternity for Professional Nurses

ATS   American Thoracic Society

AUAA   American Urological Association Allied, Inc.

AWHONN   Association of Women's Health, Obstetric, and Neonatal Nurses

CEP   Chi Eta Phi Sorority, Inc.

CGEAN   Council on Graduate Education for Administration in Nursing

CGFNS   Commission on Graduates of Foreign Nursing Schools

CHA   Catholic Health Association of the United States

CNA   Canadian Nurses' Association

DANA   Drug and Alcohol Nursing Association, Inc.

DDNA   Developmental Disabilities Nurses Association

DNA   Dermatology Nurses Association

ENA   Emergency Nurses Association

FNIF   Florence Nightingale International Foundation

FNS   Frontier Nursing Service

ICLRN   Interagency Council on Library Resources for Nursing

INS   Intravenous Nurses Society

NADONA/LTC   National Association Directors of Nursing Administration in Long Term Care

NAHC   National Association of Home Care

NAHCR   National Association for Health Care Recruitment

NAHN   National Association of Hispanic Nurses

NANDA-I   NANDA International (formerly the North American Nursing Diagnosis Association)

NANN   National Association of Neonatal Nurses

NANP   National Alliance of Nurse Practitioners

NANPRH National Association of Nurse Practitioners in Reproductive Health

NAON National Association of Orthopaedic Nurses

NAPN National Association of Physician Nurses

NAPNAP National Association of Pediatric Nurse Associates and Practitioners

NAPNES National Association for Practical Nurse Education and Service

NASN National Association of School Nurses

NBNA National Black Nurses Association, Inc.

NCCDN National Consortium of Chemical Dependency Nurses

NCF Nurses Christian Fellowship

NCSBON National Council of State Boards of Nursing, Inc.

NEF Nurses Educational Funds, Inc.

NEHW Nurses Environmental Health Watch

NFLPN National Federation of Licensed Practical Nurses, Inc.

NFNA National Flight Nurses Association

NFSNO National Federation of Specialty Nursing Organizations

NGNA National Gerontological Nursing Association

NHPA Nurse Healers Professional Associates

NLN National League for Nursing

NMCHC National Maternal and Child Health Clearinghouse

NNBA National Nurses in Business Association

NNSA National Nurses Society on Addictions

NNSDO National Nursing Staff Development Organization

NOADN National Organization for Associate Degree Nurses

NONPF National Organization of Nurse Practitioner Faculties

NOVA Nurse Organization of Veterans Affairs

NOWWN National Organization of World War Nurses

NSNA   National Student Nurses' Association
ONS   Oncology Nursing Society
RANCA   Retired Army Nurse Corps Association
RNS   Respiratory Nursing Society
SERPMHN   Society for Education and Research in
  Psychiatric Mental Health Nursing
SGNA   Society of Gastroenterology Nurses and
  Associates, Inc.
SOHEN   Society of Otorhinolaryngology and Head/
  Neck Nurses
SPN   Society of Pediatric Nurses
SRAFN   Society of Retired Air Force Nurses, Inc.
SRS   Society of Rogerian Scholars
SVN   Society for Vascular Nursing
TNS   Transcultural Nursing Society
VNAA   Visiting Nurse Associations of America

ANA STANDARDS OF PRACTICE[4]
The profession of nursing is guided by standards of
practice published by the ANA.

Assessment: The registered nurse collects and
  prioritizes comprehensive evidence-based data
  pertinent to the patient's health or situation. The
  collection of data involves the patient, family, and
  other health care providers in formulating a plan
  of care and expected outcomes.

Diagnosis: The registered nurse analyzes the
  validated assessment data to determine the
  diagnoses or issues. Validating data is completed
  in collaboration with the patient, family, and
  other health care providers.

Outcomes identification: The registered
  nurse identifies expected outcomes for a plan
  individualized to the patient or the situation.

---

[4]From White KM: *Essential guide to nursing practice,* Silver Spring,
Md., 2012, American Nurses Association.

Outcomes should be culturally appropriate, considering any associated risks, benefits, costs, current scientific evidence, and clinical expertise when formulating expected outcomes.

Planning: The registered nurse develops a plan that prescribes strategies and alternatives to attain expected outcomes. Planning is in conjunction with the patient, family, and others, as appropriate, and includes strategies that address each of the identified diagnoses or issues. Planning may include strategies for promotion and restoration of health and prevention of illness, injury, and disease. Modifications to the plan are completed based on changes in the patient health status.

Implementation: The registered nurse implements a safe and timely identified plan that includes evidence-based interventions. A plan of care should utilize available community resources and systems in collaboration with nursing colleagues and other health care professionals.

Coordination of care: The registered nurse coordinates the plan of care for the patient, including the coordination of available resources. Documentation should include all aspects of the coordination of care.

Health teaching and health promotion: The registered nurse will work to promote health and a safe environment, including providing health education that addresses such topics as healthy lifestyles, risk-reducing behaviors, developmental needs, activities of daily living, and preventive self-care.

Consultation: The registered nurse provides consultation to the identified plan in the area of the nurse's expertise. The nurse uses clinical data, theoretical frameworks, and evidence when providing consultation.

Prescriptive authority and treatment:
   The advanced practice registered nurse uses
   prescriptive authority, procedures, referrals,
   treatments, and therapies in accordance with
   state and federal laws and regulations.
Evaluation: The registered nurse conducts
   a systematic, ongoing, and criterion-based
   evaluation of the outcomes in relation to the
   structures and processes prescribed by the plan
   and the indicated timeline.

NURSING PRACTICE ACT

The Nursing Practice Act includes the statutes or laws
that mandate the Board of Nursing in each state
to outline the scope of practice and responsibilities
for registered and licensed practical/vocational
nurses and for the practice of nursing. It is the
responsibility of each nurse to know the state
statutes that govern the practice of nursing.

THE FUTURE OF NURSING[5]

- Nurses should practice to the full extent of their
  education and training.
- Nurses should achieve higher levels of education
  and training through an improved education
  system that promotes seamless academic
  progression.
- Nurses should be full partners with physicians
  and other health care professionals in redesigning
  health care in the United States.
- Effective workforce planning and policy making
  require better data collection and an improved
  information infrastructure.

---

[5]From Institute of Medicine on the Robert Wood Johnson
Foundation Initiative on the Future of Nursing: *The future of
nursing: Leading change, advancing health,* Washington, D.C., 2011,
National Academies Press.

NATIONAL PATIENT SAFETY GOALS[6]

The following are components of the 2014 National Patient Safety Goals:

1. **Accurately Identify Patients**
   Prevention: Use at least two ways to identify patients. Spell out name; have patient state his or her date of birth, address, or medical record number; use bar codes on patient ID bracelets.

2. **Accurately Administer Medications**
   Prevention: Label medicines not labeled.
   Use the Six Rights of Medication Administration.
   Make sure patients know which medicines to take when they are at home.
   Record and pass along correct information about a patient's medicines.
   Tell the patient that it is important to bring an up-to-date list of medicines every time the patient visits a doctor or is admitted for care.

3. **Take Extra Care With Patients Who Take Medicines to Thin Their Blood**
   Prevention: Ensure patient is participating in appropriate lab tests.
   Use approved organizational policy and guidelines for assessment before changes.

4. **Prevent Infection**
   Prevention: Use the hand cleaning guidelines from the Centers for Disease Control and Prevention or the World Health Organization. Use proven guidelines to prevent infections that are difficult to treat, such as infection of the blood from central lines.
   Prevent infection after surgery, including urinary tract infections that are caused by catheters.

[6]From The Joint Commission: About our standards, 2014. Retrieved from *www.jointcommission.org/standards*.

5. **Prevent Mistakes in Surgery**
   Prevention: Pause before the surgery to ensure that the correct surgery is done on the correct patient and on the correct place on the patient's body.
   Mark the correct place on the patient's body where the surgery is to be done.
6. **Use Alarms Safely**
   Prevention: Ensure that alarms on medical equipment are heard and responded to on time.
7. **Identify Patients at Risk**
   Prevention: Complete assessments of high-risk patients, including patients at risk for falls, depression, suicide, or bleeding and patients on home oxygen.

THE THREE *A*s OF HEALTH LITERACY[7]

Health literacy means the ability for each person to be able to access health care information and have the capacity to process and understand the health information needed in order to make appropriate health decisions.

1. **Accurate:** Ensure that information given to patient is correct, current, and truthful. Keep in mind reading or educational level and cultural component of each patient and adapt materials accordingly.
2. **Accessible:** Use a font size that is easy to read and add pictures. Locate material in easily accessible areas. Use a variety of delivery modes; include written, audio, and video.
3. **Actionable:** Less background information and more call to action. Include the "who, what, when, where, and how."

---

[7]From Centers for Disease Control and Prevention: CDC works for you 24-7, 2014. Retrieved from *www.cdc.gov/24-7/*.

CHAPTER 2

Values, Beliefs, and Caring

Behaviors That Demonstrate Caring (p. 16)

BEHAVIORS THAT DEMONSTRATE CARING[1]

Comforting: When comforting a patient, the nurse is able to soothe, console, or reassure a patient's fears, anxieties, and reservations.

Honesty: The personal traits of integrity, truthfulness, and straightforwardness help to make up the characteristics of honesty. Patients trust nurses and the nursing professional, knowing that nurses will be honest with them even in the midst of chaos and uncertainty.

Listening: Actively listening to patients helps to develop a trusting relationship (see Developing Good Listening Skills in Chapter 3).

Presence: Being present with patients and families at these critical times, while applying the unique knowledge and skills of professional nursing practice, demonstrates holistic care.

---

[1]From Watson J: Intentionality and caring-healing consciousness: A practice of transpersonal nursing. *Holistic Nursing Practice,* July 2002; Watson J: Jean Watson and the theory of human caring. Definition description. 2003.

Predictability: When patients trust that nurses will be consistent in providing competent care that is delivered on time and matches the patient's expectations, the patient is reassured that nursing care will be predictable and delivered as prescribed.

Consistency: Being consistent brings reliability and uniformity to a situation that otherwise might seem chaotic and overwhelming to the patient.

Patience: The quality of being able to stay focused on a task, a goal, or the needs of a patient and his or her family, even under the most difficult of situations, can help to build trust. It can be the trait of patience that helps to anchor the patient in the midst of a health care crisis. Patience can help to bring calmness to a situation that may seem to be overwhelming to others.

Responsibility: The characteristic of being accountable or answerable for one's own actions.

Teaching: Providing information so the patient can make an informed decision. Unraveling the medical terminology brings meaning and understanding.

Sensitivity: The ability to respond to the needs of others, both physical and emotional.

Touch: Touching patients is essential to good nursing care. We touch patients with the same characteristics that we speak to them, with sensitive comforting patience. The touch of a nurse is always with respect for personal privacy and culturally responsible.

Respect: The outward expression of acceptance and courtesy. Being truly respectful encompasses the ability to take into account the feelings and opinions of others in an unbiased approach.

CHAPTER 3

Communication

STEPS IN THE COMMUNICATION PROCESS

The communication process can be broken down into several commonly accepted steps.

The sender: The person or group initiating the message. This message can be verbal or nonverbal, can be ongoing or occur once, can be conscious or unconscious. Developing an effective communication style is imperative to good nursing practice (see Developing Effective Communication later in this chapter).

The receiver: The individual or group to whom the message is sent. Both the nurse and patient alternate the role of sender and receiver. When communicating to others the nurse needs to take into account the intended receiver. For example, is the communication taking place between the nurse and a child, a parent, or an older adult?

The message: This is the particular content that is sent and received. For mutual understanding, the sender and receiver must have the same basic perception of the content of the message, or be able to reach an agreement of the intent of the message, for full understanding to take place. When communicating, the nurse needs to ensure the message is clear, accurate, and meaningful to the receiver (the patient and/or family).

The channel (or medium): This is the means by which the message is sent. Some common channels are spoken voice/telephone/radio/television, written word, or electronic.

The context: This is the setting or environment in which the message is conveyed. The context can be the setting of the communication or the situation surrounding the communication. For example, communicating at a family reunion might be very different from communication in an intensive care unit.

Feedback: This is the response, generally by the receiver, as to the success of the communication. Feedback can also be specified concerning the channel, message, and context.

REASONS WE COMMUNICATE WITH PATIENTS

Sharing Information/Facts	Explaining clinic or visiting hours
Giving Advice/ Directions	A recommendation on a brand of antibiotic ointment
Teaching/Instruction	When and how to take medication The proper application for a dressing change
Consulting/Opinion	The importance and proper type of exercise

Continued

REASONS WE COMMUNICATE WITH PATIENTS—cont'd

Learning/Explanation	How to exercise properly
Setting Rules/ Guidelines	Not mixing alcohol with certain medications
Expressing Values	The importance of maintaining blood pressure (BP) within a healthy range
Expressing Creativity	Organizing medications to prevent home accidents
Expressing Philosophy	Ideas for better nutrition
Explaining Research	Lowering BP for improved cardiac function
Selling Services	Going to diabetes education offered by the facility
Networking	Offering support groups to the patient

DEVELOPING EFFECTIVE COMMUNICATION

Know what effective communication is really about. Communication is the process of transferring signals/messages between a sender and a receiver through various methods (written words, nonverbal cues, spoken words).

Have the courage to say what you think. Be confident in knowing that you can make worthwhile contributions to a conversation. Take time each day to be aware of your opinions and feelings so you can adequately convey them to others. What is important or worthwhile to one person may not be to another and may be more so to someone else.

Practice, practice, practice. Developing advanced communication skills begins with simple interactions. Communication skills can be practiced every day in settings that range from the social to the professional. New skills take time to refine, but each time you use your communication skills, you open yourself to opportunities and future partnerships.

Make eye contact. Whether you are speaking or listening, looking into the eyes of the person with whom you are conversing can make the interaction more successful. Eye contact conveys interest and encourages your partner to be interested in you in return.

Use gestures. Use gestures, including gestures with your hands and face. Make your whole body talk. Use smaller gestures for individuals and small groups. *Caution:* Don't overuse gestures!

Don't send mixed messages. Make your words, gestures, facial expressions, and tone match. Disciplining someone while smiling sends a mixed message and is therefore ineffective. If you are delivering a positive message, make your words, facial expressions, and tone also positive.

Be aware of what your body is saying. Body language can say so much more than a mouthful of words. An open stance with arms relaxed at your sides tells anyone around you that you are approachable and open to hearing what they have to say. Arms crossed and shoulders hunched, on the other hand, suggests disinterest in conversation or unwillingness to communicate. Appropriate posture and an approachable stance can make even difficult conversations flow more smoothly.

Display constructive attitudes and beliefs.
The attitudes you bring to your communication will have a huge impact on the way you compose yourself and interact with others. Choose to be honest, patient, optimistic, sincere, respectful, and accepting of others. Be sensitive to other people's feelings, and believe in others' competence.

Develop effective listening skills. Not only should one be able to speak effectively, one must listen to the other person's words and engage in communication on what the other person is speaking about. Avoid the impulse to listen only for the end of the other person's sentence so that you can blurt out the ideas or memories in your mind while the other person is speaking (see Developing Good Listening Skills later in this chapter).

DEVELOP YOUR VOICE
Frequency or Pitch
- Avoid a high or whiny voice: A high, whiny, or soft voice may be perceived to lack authority; make you sound like prey to an aggressive co-worker; or make others not take you seriously.
- Begin doing exercises to lower the pitch of your voice. Try singing, but do it an octave lower on all your favorite songs. Practice this and, after a period of time, your voice will begin to lower.

Tone
- Avoid a monotone voice. Your voice should raise and lower periodically.
- *Caution:* Try not to be *too* animated or "sing-songy."

Intensity or Volume
- Use a volume that is appropriate for the setting. Speak more softly when you are alone and close. Speak louder when you are speaking to larger groups or across larger spaces.

Speed
- *Speech rate* is the term given to the speed at which you speak. It is calculated in the number of words spoken in a minute. A normal number of words per minute (wpm) can vary significantly.
- *Instructional speech* is usually regarded as less than 110 wpm.
- *Conversational speech* falls between 130 and 200 wpm in the fast range.
- People who read books for radio or podcasts are often asked to speak at 150 to 160 wpm.

DEVELOPING GOOD LISTENING SKILLS
1. **Stop talking.** When others are talking, listen to what they are saying; do not interrupt, talk over them, or finish their sentences for them.
2. **Prepare yourself to listen.** Relax. Focus on the speaker. Put other things out of mind. Then stop and just listen.
3. **Put the speaker at ease.** Help the speaker to feel free to speak. Remember the speaker's needs and concerns. Nod or use other gestures or words to encourage the speaker to continue.
4. **Remove distractions.** Focus on what is being said: don't doodle, shuffle papers, look out the window, pick your fingernails, or similar actions.

5. **Empathize.** Try to understand the other person's point of view. Look at issues from his or her perspective. By having an open mind we can more fully empathize with the speaker. If the speaker says something that you disagree with, wait and construct an argument to counter what is said, but keep an open mind to the views and opinions of others.

6. **Be patient.** A pause, even a long pause, does not necessarily mean that the speaker has finished. Let the speaker continue in his or her own time; sometimes it takes time to formulate what to say and how to say it. Never interrupt or finish a sentence for someone.

7. **Avoid personal prejudice.** Try to be impartial. Don't become irritated and don't let the person's habits or mannerisms distract you from what the person is really saying. Focus on what is being said and try to ignore styles of delivery.

8. **Listen to the tone.** Volume and tone both add to what someone is saying. Let these help you to understand the emphasis of what is being said.

9. **Listen for ideas—not just words.** You need to get the whole picture, not just isolated bits and pieces. One of the most difficult aspects of listening is the ability to link together pieces of information to reveal the ideas of others.

10. **Wait and watch for nonverbal communication.** Gestures, facial expressions, and eye movements can all be important. Pick up the additional information being transmitted via nonverbal communication.

SPECIAL COMMUNICATION CONSIDERATIONS

Hearing impaired: Have the patient use his or her hearing aids, if available.

Limit background noise, face the patient, and get the patient's attention.

Speak clearly, and use gestures and pictures.

Give written information, keep the area well lit, and use an interpreter as needed.

Visually impaired: Alert the patient to potential hazards.

Refer to clock face numbers for placement of objects.

Use large print, Braille, audio, or e-books.

Alert the patient that someone is present with gentle physical touch.

Physically impaired: Use nonverbal cues such as head nodding or facial expressions.

Use a white board or computer tablet.

Use assistive devices familiar to the patient.

Consult with family for best communication practices.

Cognitively impaired: Use nonverbal cues such as head nodding or facial expressions.

Use short, simple words and phrases.

Observe for patient nonverbal signs.

Talk to the patient before initiating care.

Repeat statements or ideas if needed.

Rephrase, if needed, but do not change the meaning from the first statement.

Minimize visual and auditory distractions.

Consult with family for best communication practices.

Elderly patients: Get the person's attention.

Sit face to face.

Appropriate lighting is important, avoiding glare and dimly lit areas.

Maintain good eye contact while speaking slowly and clearly.

Use short, simple words and phrases.

Ask one question at a time. This may help with sensory overload.

Give the person extra time to answer.

Repeat statements or ideas if needed.

Rephrase, if needed, but do not change the meaning from the first statement.

Minimize visual and auditory distractions.

Do not shout. Remember, not everyone is deaf.

Summarize points if you are not being understood.

Expect errors or emotional outbursts in a confused person.

You may need to restart the conversation.

You may need to stop the conversation if the person is unable to communicate.

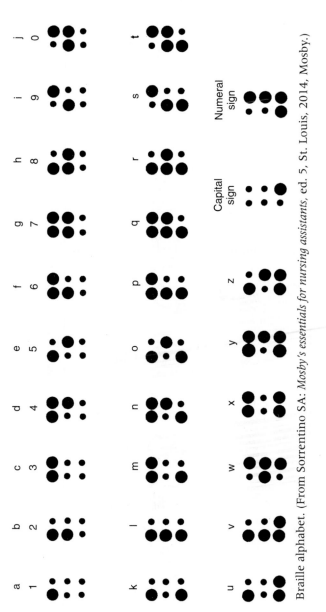

Braille alphabet. (From Sorrentino SA: *Mosby's essentials for nursing assistants*, ed. 5, St. Louis, 2014, Mosby.)

Manual alphabet

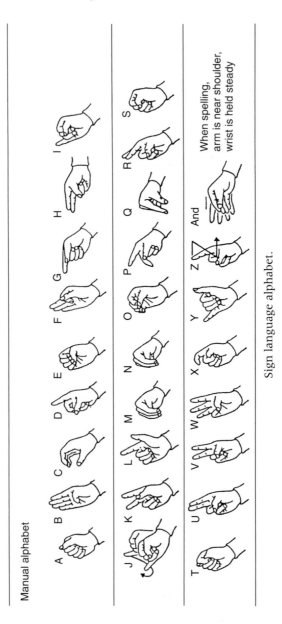

When spelling, arm is near shoulder, wrist is held steady

Sign language alphabet.

Numbers

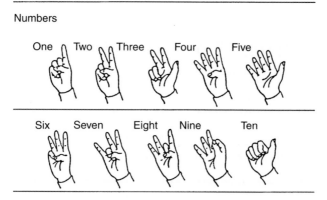

Sign language numbers.

CHAPTER 4

Critical Thinking in Nursing

CRITICAL THINKING COMPONENTS*

Critical thinking is a systemic reviewing of information obtained from observation, data collection, acquired knowledge, and personal experience. The information is evaluated for a future action. Using this definition of critical thinking is the platform on which the *nursing process* rests. The components of the critical thinking process assist the nurse with formulating a plan of care for the patient and a process by which to evaluate the outcomes.

Knowledge Review

Areas to avoid: Personal bias, illogical thinking, lack of information, closed mindedness, erroneous assumptions.

Methods to improve: Discussion with colleagues or experts, verbalization of thoughts, literature review, application of practice, concept maps, simulation, role playing.

---

*From The Foundation for Critical Thinking, 2013. Retrieved from *Criticalthinking.org*.

Information Gathering
Areas to avoid: Collecting data from too few sources or incorrect sources.
Methods to improve: Ensure data are accurate, current, and unbiased. Seek clarification for information and data not understood.

Reasoning
Areas to avoid: False assumptions, personal beliefs, making generalizations.
Methods to improve: Ask questions to clarify assumptions and personal beliefs.

Intuition
Areas to avoid: False assumptions, personal beliefs.
Methods to improve: Keep an open mind concerning alternative solutions.

Interpretation
Areas to avoid: Lack of knowledge on the subject, personal bias.
Methods to improve: Research area for understanding, to gain competence and elevate expertise. Continually reexamine data to reach best conclusion.

Validation
Areas to avoid: Problem solving without all the available facts or data.
Methods to improve: Test conclusions and generalizations before making final decision. Increase expertise by employing critical thinking skills each day.

Inductive Reasoning
Areas to avoid: Conclusions often based on observations or too few data.

Methods to improve: Test conclusions and
generalizations before making final decision.

Deductive Reasoning
Areas to avoid: Conclusions often based on
generalizations or too few data.
Methods to improve: Gather data from different
sources.

Inferences
Areas to avoid: Frequently based on assumptions
or past experiences.
Methods to improve: Reexamine data in order to
reach best conclusion.

CRITICAL THINKING IN NURSING PRACTICE
Intuition
Areas to avoid: Often based on a feeling of
knowing, rather than data.
Methods to improve: Double-check data and test
conclusions and generalizations before making
final decision.

Interpretation
Areas to avoid: Often based on own beliefs,
conceptions, experiences, and perspective.
Methods to improve: Build a broad range of
expertise from which to draw conclusions.

Analysis
Areas to avoid: Having too few data or data from
only a single source.
Methods to improve: Examine issue from
multiple sides and build expertise in analysis.

Validation

Areas to avoid: Using only subjective data to form conclusions.

Methods to improve: Validate subjective data with objective data.

Evaluation

Areas to avoid: Using one's own bias to form conclusions.

Methods to improve: Use reliable and credible sources of data.

Explanation

Areas to avoid: Using personal opinions and side comments to explain issues.

Methods to improve: Develop skills in clarity, accuracy, and precision.

Self-regulation

Areas to avoid: Making decision without reassessment of the issues.

Methods to improve: Reflect on the rationale for the conclusion.

Nursing Process

For more in-depth information on the nursing process, consult the following:

NANDA International: *Nursing diagnoses: Definitions and classification, 2012–2014,* West Sussex, England, 2012, Wiley-Blackwell.

Yoost BL, Crawford LR: *Fundamentals of nursing: Active learning for collaborative practice,* St. Louis, 2016, Mosby.

CHAPTER 5

Introduction to the Nursing Process

COMPONENTS OF THE NURSING PROCESS

The nursing process is the systematic method of critical thinking used by professional nurses to provide individualized care for patients.

Assessment: The collection of data. Patient care data are gathered through observation, interviewing the patient using standardized tools, and physical assessment.

Diagnosis: Interpretation and identification of an actual or potential problem or response to a problem.

Planning: The formation of a care plan. Prioritizes the nursing diagnoses. Identifies short- and long-term goals that are realistic, measurable, and patient focused, with specific outcome identification for evaluation purposes.

Implementation: List specific nursing interventions and treatments designed to help the patient achieve established goals or outcomes. Documentation of patient goals, interventions, and outcomes.

Evaluation: A review of effectiveness. Determines whether or not the patient's goals are met. Examines the effectiveness of interventions, and decides if the plan of care should be discontinued, continued, or revised.

CHARACTERISTICS OF THE NURSING PROCESS[1]

Complete: Each step of the nursing process should be completed for each new issue.

- Is the data collection thorough and accurate?
- Are outcomes specific and realistic for the individual patient?
- Have all of the underlying factors contributing to the patient's response to illness been adequately addressed in the plan of care?
- Could any of the nursing interventions have a negative impact on the patient?
- Does each intervention provide for patient-centered care and patient safety?
- Are there any new data that necessitate modification of the existing plan?

Dynamic: As an individual patient's condition changes, so does the way a professional nurse thinks about that patient's needs, forcing modification of earlier plans of care.

Organized: The nursing process provides a standardized method of addressing patient needs that is understood by nurses worldwide. Nurses use the nursing process as a framework for the development of individualized plans of care.

Patient centered: Designed to achieve specific outcomes, which are well defined. Patient care plans are developed to meet each individual

[1]From Yoost BL, Crawford LR: *Fundamentals of nursing: Active learning for collaborative practice,* St. Louis, 2016, Mosby.

patient's goals, not the goals of standardized patients or members of the health care team, including the nurse. Decisions regarding which nursing interventions and medical treatments to implement are made on the basis of safety and their effectiveness in meeting a patient's identified needs and desired outcomes.

Collaborative: Collaboration among several members of the health care team is often required to adequately address patient needs. In many cases, nurses incorporate orders from a primary care provider and nursing interventions with input from others, such as physical therapists, social workers, or occupational therapists, into a patient's plan of care to help alleviate patient problems and achieve established patient-centered goals and outcomes (see Critical Pathways in Chapter 8).

Adaptable: The ability to be flexible and adapt a plan of care for an individual in a hospital or receiving care in an outpatient, long-term care, or home setting. It is an equally useful method for addressing the needs of a specific population.

CHAPTER 6

Assessment

METHODS OF PATIENT ASSESSMENT

Observation: Include patient affect, clothing, personal hygiene, any obvious physical conditions, and data collected by other members of the health care team.

Patient interview: Include demographic information; data about current health concerns; perceptions of the current situation and health care; feeling of how quality of life may be affected by current situation or health status; past medical and surgical history; and any developmental, cultural, ethnic, and spiritual factors that may affect the patient.

Physical assessment: Include a head-to-toe assessment, vital signs, height and weight, and heart and lung sounds.

INTERVIEWING STRATEGIES
Open-Ended Questions

Advantages: Allow for the broadest base of information to be collected.

Disadvantages: May receive unneeded information or information that is too general.

Examples: "How can I help you?" or "Tell me more about that."

Summarizing Statements

Advantages: Rephrases patient's statements, concerns, or viewpoint.

Disadvantages: May receive limited information.

Example: "Coughing and wheezing seem to be your concerns."

Reflective Statements

Advantages: Clarify observations and can focus discussion.

Disadvantages: May limit conversation to a specific area.

Example: "You seem out of breath."

Leading Questions

Advantages: Focus questions on specific area.

Disadvantages: Limited information may be obtained.

Example: "Is your sputum green?"

Focused Questions

Advantages: Can move a conversation in a specific direction.

Disadvantages: May need additional questions to complete assessment.

Example: "Are you short of breath now?"

Clarification

Advantages: Seeks meaning to unclear information or statements.

Disadvantages: May miss important details.

Example: "When did you last take your inhaler?"

Restating
Advantages: Ensures information is clear.
Disadvantages: May limit information gathering; may need additional questions.
Example: "So you said your shortness of breath became worse yesterday?"

Encouraging
Advantages: Seeks additional information.
Disadvantages: May receive unneeded or unhelpful information.
Example: "Tell me more about your breathing."

THE PATIENT INTERVIEW[1]
Demographics: Include name, address, sex, age, birth date, marital status or significant other, religion, race, education, occupation, hobbies, significant life events.
Current situation: Reasons for seeking help or chief complaint; include annual checkup, follow-up care, second opinion, new symptoms, monitoring existing health problem(s).
History of present illness: Include location and quality of symptoms, chronology, aggravating and alleviating factors, associated symptoms, effect on lifestyle, measures used to deal with symptoms, review of body systems.
Health history: Include history of smoking, heart disease, alcohol or other drug use or abuse, surgeries, injuries, childhood diseases and vaccinations, hypertension, diabetes, arthritis, seizures, cancer, emotional problems, transfusions, drug or food allergies, perception of

[1]From Peterson V: *Clinical companion for fundamentals of nursing: Just the facts,* ed. 8, St. Louis, 2012, Mosby.

patient's health or illness, lifestyle, hygiene and eating habits, health practices.

Family medical history: Include history of heart disease, alcohol or drug use or abuse, diabetes, arthritis, cancer, emotional problems.

Medications: Prescribed, occasional use, over-the-counter, herbals; include dose, forms, and when last taken.

FUNCTIONAL ASSESSMENT[2]
Health Perceptions
General health (good, fair, poor)
Tobacco or alcohol use (how much, how long)
Recreational or prescribed medications (list)
Hygiene practices
Respiratory problems (shortness of breath)
Circulation problems (chest pain, edema, pacemaker)

Nutrition

Type of diet (list)	Enjoys snacks (yes/no, what type)
Fluid intake (types of fluids)	Fluid restriction (yes/no)
Skin (normal, dry, rash)	Teeth (own, dentures, bridge)
Weight (recent gain or loss)	Respiration and circulation

Elimination
Upper GI (nausea, vomiting, dysphagia, discomfort)
Bowels (frequency, consistency, last bowel movement, ostomy)

---

[2]From Peterson V: *Clinical companion for fundamentals of nursing: Just the facts*, ed. 8, St. Louis, 2012, Mosby.

Bladder (incontinence, dysuria, urgency, frequency, nocturia, hematuria)

Activity and Exercise
Energy level (high, normal, low)
Usual exercise and activity patterns (recent changes)
Needs assistance with (eating, bathing, dressing)
Requirements (cane, walker, wheelchair, crutches)

Sleep
Problems (falling asleep, early waking, hours per night, napping)
Methods used to facilitate sleep
Feelings on waking (fatigued, refreshed)

Cognitive
Educational level, along with learning needs and developmental age
Communication barriers (list) and memory loss (yes/no)
Reads and writes English (yes/no), or list other languages

Sensory
Hearing and vision (no problems, impaired, devices)
Pain (yes/no, how managed)

Coping and Stress
Needs (social services, financial counselor)
May need (home care, nursing home)
Coping mechanisms used by patient

Self-Perception
How illness or wellness is affecting patient
Body image or self-esteem concerns

Roles and Relationships
Significant other or emergency contacts
Primary, secondary, or tertiary roles
Role changes caused by illness or wellness
Role conflicts caused by illness or wellness

Sexuality
Last menstrual period, menopause, breast
    examination
Testicular examination
How illness may affect sexuality
How hospitalization may affect sexuality
Any questions, needs, or additional concerns

Values and Beliefs
Religious or cultural affiliation
Religious or cultural beliefs concerning health or
    illness
Holiday or food restrictions while hospitalized
Religious or cultural restrictions on medications or
    treatments
Religious or cultural rituals needed while
    hospitalized
Clergy or religious leader requested while
    hospitalized

CULTURAL ASSESSMENT[3]
Information About the Country of Origin
What is the cultural or ethnic affiliation?
In what country was the patient born?
How many years has he or she been in the United
    States?
What generation of American is the patient?

---

[3]Yoost BL, Crawford LR: *Fundamentals of nursing: Active learning for collaborative practice*, St. Louis, 2016, Mosby.

Language Needs

Does the patient need an interpreter (what language)?

Does the patient need a communication tool (language board)?

Can the patient use a telephone language line?

Cultural Practices

Are there practices or rituals that may need to be honored?

How will the illness affect cultural practices or rituals?

Cultural Supports

To whom does the patient turn for help?

How does the patient describe his or her family?

Who is the patient's main source of support, hope, or comfort?

SPIRITUAL ASSESSMENT[4]

Religious Supports

Minister, priest, rabbi, shaman, imam, other

Local clergy and telephone number

The need for church or prayer services

The need for confession, communion, or religious music

The need for a *Bible, Koran, Bhagavad-Gita,* prayer books

Religious Practices

Are there practices or rituals that may need to be honored?

Are there special religious dietary needs?

---

[4]Yoost BL, Crawford LR: *Fundamentals of nursing: Active learning for collaborative practice,* St. Louis, 2016, Mosby.

Is there a special prayer schedule that should be
  followed?
Are there special fasting rituals that should be
  followed?
How will the illness affect religious practices or
  rituals?

Religious Support Assessment Questions
Which religious supports may help your patient?
To whom does the patient turn for help?
How does the patient describe his or her family?
Who is the patient's main source of support, hope,
  or comfort?
What gives your patient's life meaning?
Does your patient believe that the illness is a
  punishment?

PHYSICAL ASSESSMENT
Appearance: Stage of development, general
  health, striking features, height, weight, behavior,
  posture, communication skills, grooming,
  hygiene.
Skin: Color, consistency, temperature, turgor,
  integrity, texture, lesions, mucous membranes.
Hair: Color, texture, amount, distribution.
Nails: Color, texture, shape, size.
Neurologic: Pupil reaction, motor and verbal
  responses, gait, reflexes, neurologic checks.
Musculoskeletal: Range of motion, gait, tone,
  posture.
Cardiovascular: Heart rate and rhythm, Homans
  sign, peripheral pulses, temperature, edema.
Respiratory: Rate, rhythm, depth, effort, quality,
  expansion, cough, breath sounds, sputum
  (production, color, and amount), tracheostomy
  size, nasal patency.

Gastrointestinal: Abdominal contour, bowel sounds, nausea, vomiting, ostomy type and care, fecal frequency, consistency, presence of blood.

Genitourinary: Urine color; character, amount, odor, ostomy.

ASSESSMENT TECHNIQUES

Inspection: By visual or auditory observation.

Auscultation: By listening to sounds with a stethoscope.

Palpation: By touching
    Fingertips: Best for texture, moisture, shape.
    Palmar surface of fingers: Best for vibration.
    Dorsum of hand: Best for temperature.

Percussion: By striking the body and assessing the sound.
    Light percussion: Best for tenderness, density.
    Sharp percussion: Best for reflexes.

CHAPTER 7

Nursing Diagnosis

TYPES OF NURSING DIAGNOSES

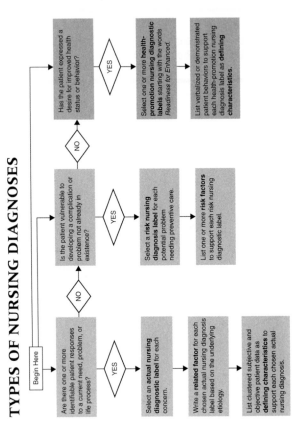

Begin Here

Are there one or more identifiable patient responses to a current need, problem, or life process?

NO → **Is the patient vulnerable to developing a complication or problem not already in existence?**

NO → **Has the patient expressed a desire for improved health status or behavior?**

YES → **Select one or more health-promotion nursing diagnostic labels starting with the words *Readiness for Enhanced*.**

→ **List verbalized or demonstrated patient behaviors to support each health-promotion nursing diagnosis label as defining characteristics.**

YES → **Select a risk nursing diagnostic label for each potential problem needing preventive care.**

→ **List one or more risk factors to support each risk nursing diagnostic label.**

YES → **Select an actual nursing diagnostic label for each concern.**

→ **Write a related factor for each chosen actual nursing diagnosis label based on the underlying etiology.**

→ **List clustered subjective and objective patient data as defining characteristics to support each chosen actual nursing diagnosis.**

THE NURSING DIAGNOSTIC PROCESS[1]
Data Collection
Areas to avoid: Cluster unrelated data, missing pertinent data, omitting key information.

Areas to improve: Through assessment and verify all data.

Data Analysis
Areas to avoid: Linking the nursing diagnosis with the cause rather than the medical issue. Basing conclusions on personal bias.

Areas to improve: Complete data, verify sources, improve assessment skills.

Underlying Issues
Areas to avoid: Data based on the cause instead of the issue.

Areas to improve: Increase understanding of pathophysiology.

Focus on One Problem or Issue
Areas to avoid: Trying to solve multiple issues with one intervention.

Areas to improve: Keep issues and solutions clear and distinct.

Patient Focused
Areas to avoid: Focusing on what the nurse needs to "get done."

Areas to improve: Focus only on what the patient needs to achieve.

---

[1]Yoost BL, Crawford LR: *Fundamentals of nursing: Active learning for collaborative practice*, St. Louis, 2016, Mosby.

CHAPTER 8

Planning

GOAL CRITERIA[1]

Patient centered: Reflects the patient's needs, choices, behavior, and responses.

  Example: Patient will begin walking twice each week for weight loss.

Mutually agreed: Increases the patient's motivation and cooperation.

  Example: Patient agrees to increase exercise program to twice each week.

Singular: Should address only one need, behavior, or response.

  Example: Patient will switch from regular soda to diet soda for weight loss.

Observable: Must be able to observe if change takes place in a patient's status.

  Example: Patient will walk with spouse as part of exercise program.

Achievable: Goals must be obtainable for the patient to be successful.

---

[1]From Potter PA, Perry AG: *Fundamentals of nursing*, ed. 8, St. Louis, 2012, Mosby.

Example: Patient will begin with walking once a
week for 2 weeks, then increase to twice each
week on week 3.
Measurable: Should measure the patient's progress
toward the stated goal; terms describing quality,
quantity, frequency, length, or weight allow you
to evaluate outcomes precisely.
Example: Patient will track in weekly journal
the frequency and distance walked each week.
Realistic: Provide patient a sense of hope that
increases motivation and cooperation.
Example: Patient will begin with ¼ mile (two
to three blocks) distance for each walk, then
increase the distance to 1 mile over the
timeframe of 6 months.
Time limited: Timeframes assist in determining
if the patient is making progress and promote
accountability in the delivery and management of
nursing care.
Example: Patient will call the clinic in 1 month
to update goals.

INDIVIDUALIZING PATIENT CARE[2]

Individualizing a patient's plan of care begins with
an application of the nursing process; a thorough
assessment of the patient, including medical and
nursing diagnoses and goals to be reached; an
analysis of the current data; and critical judgment
of the abilities and wishes of the patient. To meet
each patient's needs, care plans are individualized
through the following considerations.
Patient situation, age, and gender: Tailor the
plan of care, taking into account a younger versus

---

[2]Yoost BL, Crawford LR: *Fundamentals of nursing: Active learning for
collaborative practice*, St. Louis, 2016, Mosby.

elderly patient, and how the current health situation has altered the patient's abilities.

Disabilities: Ensure that the patient is physically able to complete the plan of care. For example, someone wearing a cast may not be able to begin a walking regimen for weight loss until the cast has been removed. Asking a patient to learn about the health care condition when a patient is unable to read, or unable to read English, will cause the patient to be unsuccessful.

Health literacy: Ensure patient education materials are at a reading level appropriate for the patient and accessible to patients and family (see The Three *A*s of Health Literacy in Chapter 1).

Cultural or religious traditions and values: Ensure that the plan of care takes into account the traditions and rituals of the patient. For example, expecting a patient to perform health care tasks on days of the week considered holy by the patient, or performing tasks to members of the opposite sex, might be considered off-limits (see Cultural and Spiritual Assessments in Chapter 6).

Patient expectations: Ensure that the patient care plan and its goals are patient centered and agreed upon by the patient (see Goal Criteria earlier in this chapter). Asking what the patient wants and needs is the first step to a successful outcome. For example, ask if the patient wants to return directly home after hospitalization or if the patient would rather go to a skilled care facility or temporarily remain with family.

Support system: Ensuring that the patient has a support system in place before discharge can assist in the successfulness of the transition from hospital to home.

Personal preferences: Implement patient education based on the preference of each patient (see Patient Education Assessment Questions in Chapter 13).

DEVELOPMENT OF A PATIENT CARE PLAN

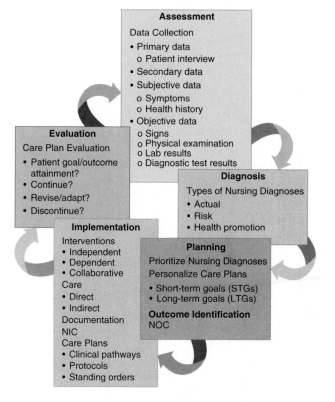

Assessment

Data Collection
- Primary data
  o Patient interview
- Secondary data
- Subjective data
  o Symptoms
  o Health history
- Objective data
  o Signs
  o Physical examination
  o Lab results
  o Diagnostic test results

Diagnosis

Types of Nursing Diagnoses
- Actual
- Risk
- Health promotion

Planning

Prioritize Nursing Diagnoses
Personalize Care Plans
- Short-term goals (STGs)
- Long-term goals (LTGs)

Outcome Identification
NOC

Implementation

Interventions
- Independent
- Dependent
- Collaborative
Care
- Direct
- Indirect
Documentation
NIC
Care Plans
- Clinical pathways
- Protocols
- Standing orders

Evaluation

Care Plan Evaluation
- Patient goal/outcome attainment?
- Continue?
- Revise/adapt?
- Discontinue?

PATIENT CARE PLAN COMPONENTS

Care Components	Patient Outcome	Nursing Intervention	Evaluation
List the diagnosis	List the goals	List the interventions	—
Related to the specific problem	Each action should have an outcome	Actions per nurse	Can the patient accomplish the goals?
Secondary to the medical diagnosis	Consider the time needed to achieve the goals	Actions per patient	Did the patient accomplish the goals?
As manifested by the signs and symptoms	Consider individualizing the care plan	Individualize interventions	Did the symptoms resolve?

PRIORITIZATION OF PATIENT NEEDS

Level Category (Needs)	Examples of Data
Physiologic	Airway patency, breathing, circulation, oxygen level, nutrition, fluid intake, body temperature regulation, warmth, elimination, shelter, sexuality, infection, pain level.
Safety and Security	Physical safety (falls and drug side effects); psychological security (knowledge of routines and procedures, bedtime rituals, fear of isolation and dependence needs).
Love and Belonging	Compassion of care provider, information from family and significant others, strength of support system.
Self-Esteem	Changes in body image (injury, surgery, puberty); changes in self-concept (ability to perform usual role functions); pride in abilities.
Self-Actualization	Goal attainment, autonomy, motivation, problem-solving abilities, ability to provide and accept help, feeling of accomplishment, desired roles.

Source: Maslow AH: *Motivation and personality,* ed. 2, New York, 1970, Harper & Row.

CRITICAL PATHWAYS[3]

Critical pathways incorporate a multidisciplinary approach to patient care. When developing a patient's plan of care through the use of critical pathways, consider some of the following questions:

Medicine: Which medical treatments will be recommended? How will these treatments affect the plan of care and the patient's outcomes? How will the prognosis affect the plan of care and the patient's outcomes?

Pharmacy: What medications will be prescribed? How will the medications affect the plan of care and the patient's outcomes?

Therapy: Will physical or occupational therapy be prescribed? How will therapy affect the plan of care and the patient's outcomes? What kind of discharge planning is needed? When in the patient's course of treatment should discharge planning begin? How will the discharge plans affect the plan of care and the patient's outcomes?

Social work: Will financial, social, or family services be needed for the patient? How will these services affect the plan of care and the patient's outcomes?

Chaplain: Will emotional or spiritual support be needed for the patient? How will this support affect the plan of care and the patient's outcomes?

[3]From Peterson V: *Clinical companion for fundamentals of nursing: Just the facts,* ed. 8, St. Louis, 2012, Mosby.

CHAPTER 9

Implementation and Evaluation

DIRECT/INDIRECT CARE
- **Direct care** refers to interventions that are carried out by having personal contact with patients. *Examples:* cleaning an incision, administering an injection, reassessment, assisting with activities of daily living, counseling, teaching.
- **Indirect care** includes nursing interventions performed to benefit patients, without face-to-face nurse-patient contact. *Examples:* change-of-shift report, communication and collaboration with members of the interdisciplinary health care team, ensuring availability of needed equipment, referrals, research, delegation.

TYPES OF INTERVENTIONS
- **Independent nursing interventions** are tasks within the nursing scope of practice that the nurse may undertake without a physician or primary care provider (PCP) order. *Examples:* determining what nursing interventions

to include in a patient's plan of care and prioritizing that care, repositioning a patient in bed, performing oral hygiene, and providing emotional support through active listening.

- **Dependent nursing interventions** are tasks that the nurse undertakes that are within the nursing scope of practice but require the order of a physician or PCP to implement. *Example:* administering medications or oxygen to a patient.
- **Collaborative interventions** may involve the expertise of different members of the health care team.

THE EVALUATION PROCESS
- Determines if patient goals are met.
- Determines if new data have been identified since care began that should be taken into consideration.
- Examines the extent to which interventions affected patient outcomes.
- Evidence-based practices should be used to formulate a care plan and to help evaluate the effectiveness and outcomes.
- Does the care plan need to be modified in response to patient changes?
- Based on the patient's response to the implemented interventions, should the plan of care be continued, revised, or discontinued?

SAFE PRACTICE ALERTS!
- Before implementing any patient interventions, the nurse must check patient identity using two methods. This critical safety step prevents interventions from being performed on the wrong person.

- Make sure the patient is alert and oriented before conducting a health history or asking the patient to make significant health care decisions.
- Remember that following protocols or implementing standing orders still requires critical thinking and use of the nursing process to determine the applicability of interventions in specific patient care circumstances.
- Blindly following critical pathways, protocols, or standing orders is contraindicated in all nursing care situations.

Nursing Practice

For more in-depth information on nursing practice, consult the following:

Institute for Healthcare Improvement. 2014. Retrieved from *www.ihi.org/Pages/default.aspx*.

NANDA International: *Nursing diagnoses: Definitions and classification, 2012–2014*, West Sussex, England, 2012, Wiley-Blackwell.

Office of Disease Prevention and Health Promotion: *Healthy People 2020*, 2014. Retrieved from *www.healthypeople.gov*.

Yoost BL, Crawford LR: *Fundamentals of nursing: Active learning for collaborative practice,* St. Louis, 2016, Mosby.

CHAPTER 10

Documentation, Electronic Health Records, and Reporting

CHARTING

Source-oriented records: Include admission sheet, physicians' orders, history, nurses' notes, tests, and reports.

Problem-oriented records: Include database, problem list, physicians' orders, care plans, and progress notes.

COMPONENTS OF DOCUMENTATION

Expected nursing documentation includes a nursing assessment, care plan, interventions, teaching, the patient's outcomes or response to care, and assessment of ability to manage after discharge.

- Be factual, without exaggeration or understatement.
- Be nonjudgmental, without personal opinions or personal bias.
- Be accurate with medical terminology; use correct spelling and proper grammar.
- Be complete and use correct sequencing of events as they happened.
- Be concise, avoiding unneeded words or phrases.
- Document as soon as possible after assessment, interventions, condition changes, or evaluation.
- Each entry must include the date, time, and signature with credentials of the person.
- Do not erase or alter with correction fluid, because documentation may be used in legal action.
- Only approved abbreviations may be used (see Unacceptable Abbreviations later in this chapter).

DOCUMENTATION FORMATS

Use the approved documentation formats per organizational policy.

APIE (assessment, problem, intervention, evaluation)
AIR (assessment, intervention, results)
CBE (charting by exception)
DAR (data, action, response)
Flow sheet notes or data written in a graph format
Narrative notes written in a paragraph form
PIE (problem, intervention, evaluation)
SOAP (subjective data, objective data, assessment, plan)
SOAPIE (subjective data, objective data, assessment, plan, intervention, evaluation)

SOAPIER (subjective data, objective data, assessment, plan, intervention, evaluation, results)

DOCUMENTATION FORMS

Flow sheets: Document care and observations recorded on a regular basis. May be converted to a graph.

Medication Administration Record (MAR): Lists ordered medications, dosage, administration times, signature.

Bar-coded medication administration: Uses portable scanner to scan patient's wristband and medication to be given. Tracks medications given, held, refused, or due.

Kardex: Documents patient information, such as patient demographic information.

Admission and discharge: Include patient history, medication reconciliation, discharge planning needs, status at discharge, patient education, and referrals.

Pediatric growth charts: Usually completed for height, weight, and head and chest circumference.

Incident reports: Record facts of unexpected events; not generally part of medical record.

Presurgery checklist: Include patient name, list of valuables, list of prostheses and if they have been removed before surgery, preop labs, preop scrub, notation of the signed consent form, and where the family will be during surgery.

Postoperative checklist: Type of surgery and anesthetic, complications, transfusions, current physical assessment, vital signs, dressing location and condition, postoperative orders, notification of family.

Blood administration checklist: Patient's name, date of birth, blood type, time and duration of transfusion, premedications, type of tubing and fluids for flushing, vital signs.

UNACCEPTABLE ABBREVIATIONS

Old Abbreviations	Consider Using
AD	Right ear or R-ear
AS	Left ear or L-ear
AU	Both ears
OD	Right eye or R-eye
OS	Left eye or L-eye
OU	Both eyes
QD (qd)	Each day or daily
QID (qid)	4× each day or 4× daily
QOD (qod)	Every other day
Qh (qh)	Every or each hour
QW (qw)	Every or each week
Q×H (q×h)	4× an hour
BIW	Twice per week
TIW	Three time per week
MS, MSO_4, $MgSO_4$	Spell out morphine or magnesium
U	Units
IU (iu)	International units
μg	Micrograms
×3d	3×each day or 3×daily
Cc	mL
< >	Spell out: less than, greater than
. .. ...	1, 2, 3
⊤ ⊤⊤ ⊤⊤⊤ ♀ ♀♀ ♀♀♀	One, two, three

From The Joint Commission: Do Not Use" List of Abbreviations, 2012. The Joint Commission (TJC). 2012; the National Pharmacy Association; and the 2014 Patient Safety Fact Sheets. Retrieved from *www.jointcommission.org/about_us/patient_safety_fact_sheets.aspx*.

PREFIXES

a-, an- absent
ab- away from
ad- to or toward
aer- air
angio- blood vessel
ante- before
arteri- artery
aud- ear
bi- two
brady- slow
cardi- heart
cephal- head
cerebro- brain
chole- gallbladder
chondr- cartilage
cirrho- yellow
co-, con- with, together
colo- colon
contra- opposing
cost- rib
cran- head
crani- skull
cyano- blue
cysto- liquid-filled urinary bladder
dactyl- fingers or toes
de- down, from
dent(o)- teeth
derma- skin
dis- away, separate
dys- bad, difficult
e- without
encephala- brain
endo- within, inside
enter- intestines
epi- on, over
erythro- red

ex-, extra- outside of
gastr- stomach
glycol- sugar
hem- blood
hemato- blood
hemi- one half
hepat- liver
hyper- above, beyond
hypo- beneath, below
ileo- ileum
ili- ilium
inter- between
intra-, intro- within
leuko- white
lingu- tongue
lip- fat
litho- stone
macro- large
mal- bad
mega- large
melano- black
mesi-, meso- middle
meta- change
micro- small
mono- one
multi- many
my- muscle
myel- bone marrow
myelo- spinal cord
neo- new, recent
nephr- kidney
neuro- nervous system
ophthalm- eye
osteo- bone
ot- ear
par- near
para- beside, near

per- through
peri- around
phag- eat
phleg- vein
pneum- lung
polio- gray
poly- many
post- after
pre-, pro- before
proct- rectal
psycho- the mind
re- back
ren- kidney

retro- back
rhin-, rhino- nose
semi- half
splen- spleen
spondyl- spinal cord
sub- below
super-, supra- above
tachy- fast
tetra- four
tri- three
uni- one
vascular- blood vessel
venous- vein

SUFFIXES

-ac, -al pertaining to
-algia pain
-ate, -ize use, subject
-cele protrusion
-centesis puncture to
   remove fluid
-cle, -cule small
-cyte cell
-dynia pain
-ectomy removal
-emesis vomit
-emia blood
-ent, -er, -ist person
-esis, -tion condition
-genic origin
-gram, -graphy written
   record
-graph instrument that
   records
-ia, -ism, -ity condition
-iasis presence of
-ible, -ile capable

-itis inflammation
-logy study of
-megaly enlargement
-ola, -ole small
-oma tumor
-osis, -sis abnormal
-ostomy opening
-ous, -tic pertaining to
-oxia oxygen
-pathy disease
-penia deficiency of
-pexy, -pexis fixation
-phagia, -phagy eating
-phobia fear
-plasty surgical shaping
-pnea breathing
-ptosis prolapse, down
-rrhage excessive flow
-rrhage, -rrhagia
   suturing
-rrhea flow
-rrhexis suture

-scope examination instrument
-scopy examination
-stomy surgical opening
-tic relating to
-tion condition

-tome instrument
-tomy incision
-ule small
-ulum small
-ulus small
-uria urine

BODY FLUIDS

aqua- water
chol(e)- bile
dacry(o)- tears
galact(o)- milk
hem(a)- blood
hemat(o)- blood
hydro- water
lacrima- tears
mucus secretions from membranes

plasm- blood
ptyal(o)- saliva
pus liquid inflammation
sangui- blood
sanguin(o)- very bloody
serum clear portion of blood
urea-, uro- urine

BODY SUBSTANCES AND CHEMICALS

adip(o)- fat
amyl(o)- starch
cerumen earwax
collagen connective tissue
ele(o)-, ole(o)- oil
ferrum iron
glyc(o)- sugar
hal(o)- salt
hyal(o)- translucent

lapis stone
lip(o)- lipid fat, fatty
lith(o)- stone or calculus
mel(i)- honey, sugar
natrium sodium
petrous stony hardness
sabum sebaceous gland
sacchar(o)- sugar
sal- salt

COLORS

albus white
chlor(o)- green
chrom(o)- color
cirrhos- orange, yellow
cyan(o)- blue

erythr(o)- red
leuc(o)- white
lutein yellow
melan(o)- black
poli(o)- gray

rhod(o)- red

ruber- red

rubor red

xanth(o)- yellow

MEDICAL SYMBOLS

♀ standing

♀⌐ sitting

○- lying

↑ increasing

↓ decreasing

L left

R right

♀ female

♂ male

℥ dram

℥ ounce

° degree

′ minute

°**C** degrees Celsius or centigrade

°**F** degrees Fahrenheit

® registered trademark

* birth

⊤ death

Θ normal

× times

= equal to

≈ approximately

ø none or no

→ leading to

@ at

number

″ seconds

μ**g** microgram

μ**m** micrometer

ᵛ systolic blood pressure

ᴧ diastolic blood pressure

BODY REGIONS

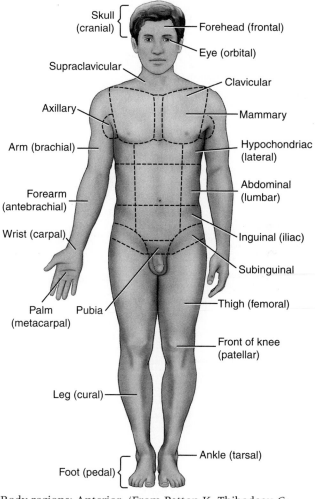

Body regions: Anterior. (From Patton K, Thibodeau G: *Structure and function of the human body,* ed. 14, St. Louis, 2012, Mosby.)

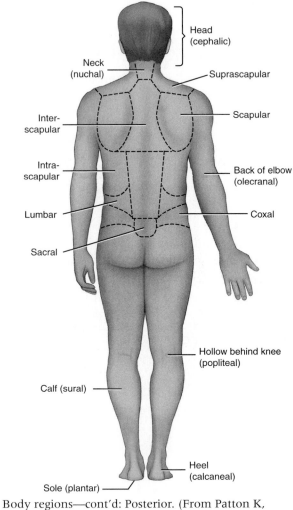

Head
(cephalic)

Neck
(nuchal)

Suprascapular

Inter-
scapular

Scapular

Intra-
scapular

Back of elbow
(olecranal)

Lumbar

Coxal

Sacral

Hollow behind knee
(popliteal)

Calf (sural)

Heel
(calcaneal)

Sole (plantar)

Body regions—cont'd: Posterior. (From Patton K,
Thibodeau G: *Structure and function of the human body,* ed.
14, St. Louis, 2012, Mosby.)

BODY CAVITIES

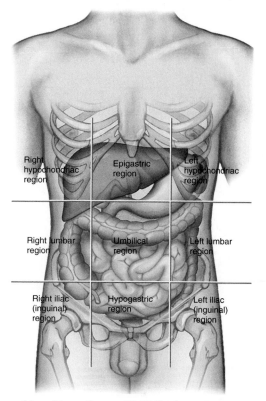

Body cavities. (From Patton K, Thibodeau G: *Structure and function of the human body,* ed. 14, St. Louis, 2012, Mosby.)

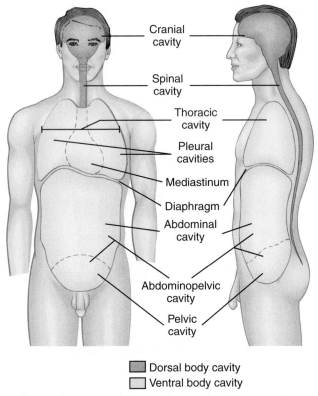

Cranial cavity

Spinal cavity

Thoracic cavity

Pleural cavities

Mediastinum

Diaphragm

Abdominal cavity

Abdominopelvic cavity

Pelvic cavity

Dorsal body cavity
Ventral body cavity

Body cavities—cont'd. (From Patton K, Thibodeau G: *Structure and function of the human body,* ed. 14, St. Louis, 2012, Mosby.)

DIRECTIONS AND PLANES

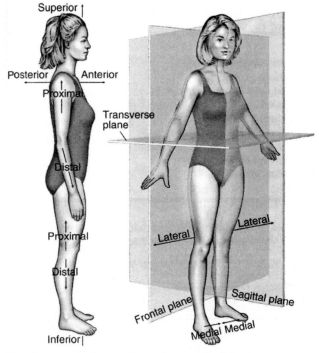

Directions and planes. (From Patton K, Thibodeau G: *Structure and function of the human body,* ed. 14, St. Louis, 2012, Mosby.)

ELEMENTS OF A GOOD HAND-OFF REPORT[1]

The transfer of care (hand-off) from one health care professional to another is a daily and important part of nursing care. The elements of

---

[1]From Institute for Healthcare Improvement, 2014. Retrieved from *www.ihi.org/Pages/default.aspx*.

a good hand-off report will differ depending on the situation, the institution, and the level of professional giving and receiving the hand-off. The **SBAR** (**S**ituation, **B**ackground, **A**ssessment, and **R**ecommendation) is a standardized systematic approach in transferring patient care.

Situation: Including the introduction of the patient (patient's name, age, date of birth, address). What is happening at the present time?

Background: What are the circumstances leading up to this situation? Any changes in the patient's status and vital signs?

Assessment: What do I think the problem is? Based on the physical, emotional, and vital sign assessment, what is the issue that needs the most immediate attention?

Recommendation: What should we do to correct the problem? Allow for questions and clarification of any information.

CHANGE-OF-SHIFT REPORT

The outgoing nurse discusses with the oncoming nurse the condition of the patient and any changes that have occurred to the patient during the shift. The guidelines or policy of the structure and content for the change-of-shift report may vary by institution. It is the responsibility of all nurses to know the policy of the organization in which they work.

Basic components may include the following:

- Patient's name, age, room number, and diagnosis
- Reason for admission, date, and type of surgery, if applicable
- Significant changes during the shift and during the past 24 hours
- Tests and procedures during the previous shift
- Tests and procedures for the upcoming shift

- Important laboratory data, current physical and emotional assessments
- Vital signs if abnormal, intake and output, IV fluid status
- Activity during the past shift
- Discharge plans
- Updated changes or effectiveness of care plan on appropriate document

CHAPTER 11

Ethical and Legal Considerations

THE PATIENT'S CHART (PAPER CHART)

- The patient's chart is a legal document that can be called as evidence in a legal action.
- Be complete, concise, legible, and accurate.
- Use ink, sign all charting, cross out errors with a single line, and initial.
- Do not erase or used fluid correction.
- Do not leave spaces.
- Use standard abbreviations and proper medical terminology.
- Include date, time, and credentials.
- Use proper grammar and accurate spelling.
- Do not place a facilities incident report in the patient's chart.

ELECTRONIC MEDICAL RECORD (EMR)

- An electronic medical record (EMR) is a legal document that can be called as evidence in a legal action.
- Document using ONLY your username and password.
- Do NOT document using someone else's username and password.
- Double-check to ensure that documentation appears in the correct EMR.
- Use standard abbreviations and proper terminology.
- Use proper grammar and accurate spelling.
- Know the organizational policies for releasing information.
- Follow organizational policy for electronic signatures.
- Follow all organizational confidentiality policies regarding the EMR.

According to the Health Insurance Portability and Accountability Act (HIPAA), the patient owns the information contained within the EMR and has a right to view the originals and to obtain copies under law. However, the actual physical copy of the medical record is the legal property of the health care facility or institution. Health care workers need to know and follow the organizational policies for releasing information to patients.

HIPAA CONSIDERATIONS[1]

Privacy: Allows an individual to control the sharing of personal information by requiring predisclosure authorization.

---

[1]From Yoost BL, Crawford LR: *Fundamentals of nursing: Active learning for collaborative practice,* St. Louis, 2016, Mosby.

Confidentiality: Limits disclosure of private information to only authorized persons.

Procedural concerns: Patients must be offered or have access to a notice of their rights.

- Patient names cannot be posted or released.
- Discussion of patient information cannot be held in public-access areas, and discussions in nursing areas must be held in soft voices.
- Using a camera and/or recorder or not concealing patient information while preparing school assignments is considered a violation of the act, resulting in penalties.
- Paper or electronic charts cannot be visible or left in an open, public-access area.
- Fax transmissions have parameters to protect privacy.
- Electronic medical records (EMRs) must be password protected with access given only to those who need it to provide care or those who the patient has authorized.
- Personnel must log off computers when finished working with patient records. Computers must have the protection of an automatic log-off after a certain period of inactivity.
- Passwords should never be shared.
- Patient information should never be e-mailed or faxed unless the transmission is encrypted and special arrangements have been made for receiving the data.
- Firewalls and other Internet technology protections should be installed to prevent unwarranted intrusions and identity theft.

Documentation concerns: Patients' rights include the following:

- Obtaining, viewing, and/or updating a copy of their own medical records.

- Obtaining information regarding HIPAA and how the facility will use personal information that is collected and requesting variants on those uses.
- Choosing how to receive information and education about their health.
- Paper documentation should not be thrown in the trash; it must be shredded. This includes scrap paper and report memorandums.

PROFESSIONAL NURSING BEHAVIOR

The National Council of State Boards of Nursing recognizes specific nurse behaviors as indicating a potential for professional boundary violations, including the following:
- Engaging in excessive self-disclosure of personal information to a patient.
- Keeping secrets with a patient; limiting others from conversation and patient information.
- Spending excessive amounts of time with one patient, unless medically necessary.
- Acting as if a patient is a family member or close personal friend.
- Failing to protect the patient from inappropriate sexual involvement with the nurse.

INFORMED CONSENT[2]

In general, informed consent assumes that a patient is legally able to make his or her own decisions. For informed consent to take place, the information that is given must be understood. States have developed informed consent laws to govern certain types of communication between health providers and patients. These laws vary from state to state; however, the laws list the types of

[2]From Yoost BL, Crawford LR: *Fundamentals of nursing: Active learning for collaborative practice,* St. Louis, 2016, Mosby.

information that patients must be given so they can make an informed decision about having medical care, diagnostic tests, or treatment. Some of the components of the informed consent form include the following:

- Name of hospital, facility, organization, or agency
- Name of procedure(s) or treatment(s)
- Name of practitioner performing the procedure
- Name of practitioner who conducted the informed consent
- Statement of procedure, risks, benefits, and alternatives
- Listing of the risks
- Signature of patient or legal representative
- Date of patient signature
- Time of day of patient signature
- Signature of witness
- Date and time of day of witness signature

ADVANCE DIRECTIVES

1. **Living will** (also known as personal directive, advance directive, or advance decision): Specifies the treatment a person wishes to receive if the person is no longer able to make decisions because of illness or incapacity.
2. **Durable power of attorney:** Allows a designated person to make legal decisions on behalf of a person not able to make independent legal decisions.
3. **Health care proxy:** Specifies who is to make health care decisions for an individual unable to make his or her own decisions.
4. **Five wishes:** A national (U.S.) advance directive created by the nonprofit organization Aging with Dignity. This document combines a living will and health care power of attorney in addition to addressing matters of comfort care and spirituality.

Wishes 1 and 2 are both legal documents.
Once signed, they meet the legal requirements for
an advance directive in many states. Wishes 3, 4,
and 5 address matters of comfort care, spirituality,
forgiveness, and final wishes.

Wish 1: Lists the person who will make care
decisions.

Wish 2: Lists the kind of medical treatment the
person wants and does not want.

Wish 3: Explains how comfortable the person
wishes to be or what comfort measures the
person wants.

Wish 4: Explains how and where the person wishes
to be treated, such as wanting to remain at home,
or whether praying, singing, and so forth should
be done at the person's bedside.

Wish 5: Explains any final wishes regarding the
death, funeral, or memorial plans.

Each of these advance directive documents serves
a unique and valuable role. Individuals should
consider reviewing several document styles to
ensure that they complete the document that best
meets their personal needs.

CHAPTER 12

Leadership and Management

PRINCIPLES OF DELEGATION[1]

The decision of whether or not to delegate is based on the professional nurse's clinical judgment and must take into account the condition of the patient, the competence of the person to whom the tasks are being delegated, and the degree of supervision that will be required of the registered nurse (RN).

- RN takes responsibility and accountability for his or her own nursing practice.
- RN determines the appropriate utilization of any assistant involved in providing direct patient care.
- RN may delegate components of nursing care but does not delegate the nursing process itself.
- RN delegates only those tasks for which the other health care worker has the knowledge and skill to perform.
- RN verifies comprehension with the unlicensed assistive personnel (UAP) and that the UAP

---

[1]From The Joint Statement on Delegation American Nurses Association (ANA) and the National Council of State Boards of Nursing (NCSBN).

accepts the delegation and the responsibility that accompanies it.

- UAPs should have the opportunity to ask questions and/or get clarification of expectations.
- RN uses the Five Rights of Delegation to be sure that the delegation or assignment is:
  - The right task
  - Under the right circumstances
  - To the right person
  - With the right directions and communication
  - Under the right supervision and evaluation

THE FIVE RIGHTS OF DELEGATION[2]

The Right Task: Appropriate delegation activities are identified for specific client(s). The task requires no nursing judgment with outcomes that are reasonably predictable. The task does not require complex observations or critical decisions without repeated nursing assessments.

The Right Circumstance: Assess health status of individual client(s), analyze the data, and identify client-specific goals and nursing care needs. Appropriate patient setting, available resources, and other relevant factors are considered. There is no need to alter the procedure for completing the task.

To the Right Person: Verify and identify UAP's competency on an individual and client-specific basis.

With the Right Directions: Clear, concise description of the task, including its objective,

---

[2]From The Joint Statement on Delegation American Nurses Association (ANA) and the National Council of State Boards of Nursing (NCSBN): *The consequences of delegating the task are not a risk to the patient* (Ohio Board of Nursing, 2009; Carr & Pearson, 2005).

limits, and expectations. Specific communication includes specific data to be collected and method and timelines for reporting, specific activities to be performed and any client-specific instruction and limitation, and the expected results or potential complications and timelines for communicating such information.

Under the Right Supervision: Appropriate monitoring, evaluation, intervention, and feedback. Intervene if necessary, and ensure proper documentation.

CHAPTER 13

Health Literacy and Patient Education

HEALTH LITERACY

Health literacy is the degree to which individuals have the capacity to obtain, process, and understand basic health information needed to make appropriate health decisions and identify services needed to prevent or treat illness.

EXPECTED PATIENT COMPETENCIES FOR HEALTH LITERACY: *HEALTHY PEOPLE 2020*[1]

- Read and identify credible health information for specific health care issues.
- Understand numbers in the context of the patient's health care.
- Make appointments.
- Fill out forms.
- Gather health records and ask appropriate questions of physicians.

---

[1]From Office of Disease Prevention and Health Promotion: *Healthy People 2020,* 2014. Retrieved from *www.healthypeople.gov.*

- Advocate for appropriate care.
- Navigate complex insurance and financial assistance programs.
- Use technology to access information and services.

ASSESSMENT QUESTIONS RELATED TO PATIENT EDUCATION[2]

- Who will be taking care of you?
- Who do we need to educate?
- What do you already know about your diagnosis or care of this condition?
- What is your preferred language?
- Do you have access to the Internet?
- What is the highest grade level that you completed in school?
- Do you read the local newspaper? Books? Magazines?
- What do you hope to learn from our teaching sessions?
- What information do you feel is most important?
- Have you ever had instruction on this subject? (If so, ask for details.)
- How do you feel you learn best? By watching and doing? By reading?
- Do you have any difficulty with hearing or vision?
- Do you need glasses for reading?
- Are there barriers that may prevent you from learning?

[2]From Yoost BL, Crawford LR: *Fundamentals of nursing: Active learning for collaborative practice,* St. Louis, 2016, Mosby.

CHAPTER 14

Health and Wellness

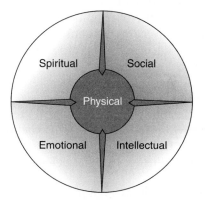

Physical	Fitness. Nutrition. Medical self-care. Control of substance abuse.
Emotional	Care for emotional crisis. Stress management.
Social	Communities. Families. Friends.
Intellectual	Educational. Achievement. Career development.
Spiritual	Love. Hope. Charity.

Dimensions of optimal health. (Reprinted with permission from *American Journal of Health Promotion*.)

LEVELS OF PREVENTION

- **Primary prevention:** Keep disease from occurring.
  - *Goal:* Modify risk factors.
  - *Example:* Lifestyle changes, improved nutrition or increased exercise.
- **Secondary prevention:** Disease is detectable by medical tests.
  - *Goal:* Early detection and diagnosis of illness.
  - *Example:* Screening tests such as mammograms or fecal occult blood testing.
- **Tertiary prevention:** Treatment or rehabilitation care of condition.
  - *Goal:* Reduce complications and disability.
  - *Example:* Cardiac rehabilitation or physical therapy.

SAFE PRACTICE ALERTS!

- Do not use abbreviations or medical terminology when providing patients with instructions.
- Remember to follow up with unlicensed assistive personnel to ensure that the delegated task is complete.
- Medications administered must be documented immediately to avoid confusion about what has been given and the possibility of double dosing.
- Documentation should occur on a timely basis. Bedside and mobile computers enable real-time charting.
- Sign-on and password codes for access to an electronic health record system must never be shared with anyone.

Nursing Assessment

For more in-depth information on nursing assessment, consult the following:

Yoost BL, Crawford LR: *Fundamentals of nursing: Active learning for collaborative practice,* St. Louis, 2016, Mosby.

CHAPTER 15

Human Development

AGE AND DEVELOPMENTAL STAGES

	Erikson (Psychosocial)	Piaget (Cognitive)	Kohlberg (Learning)
Infant	*Trust vs. mistrust:* Dependent on others to meet needs	*Sensorimotor:* Actions are reflexive in nature	*Preconventional:* No sense of "good" or "bad" behavior
Toddler	*Autonomy vs. shame:* Beginning to assert authority over own actions	*Sensorimotor:* Realizes own actions cause reactions in others	*Preconventional:* Behavior based on rules imposed by others, motivation is to avoid punishment
Preschool	*Initiative vs. guilt:* Focus is on energetic learning	*Preoperational:* Preconceptual (2-4 yr): Egocentric thought processes, magical thinking	*Preconventional:* Motivation for behavior is to avoid punishment Does not understand reasons for the rules
		Intuitive thought (4-7 yr): Beginning sense of others' perspectives	

Continued

AGE AND DEVELOPMENTAL STAGES—cont'd

	Erikson (Psychosocial)	Piaget (Cognitive)	Kohlberg (Learning)
School-age	*Industry vs. inferiority:* Eager to develop skills, motivated to complete tasks	*Concrete operations:* Uses thought processes to experience events Able to see another's viewpoints and classify objects Concept of conservation is mastered	*Conventional level:* After age 7, able to judge actions by intentions rather than consequences
Adolescent	*Identity vs. confusion:* Focuses on who they are and who they want to become	*Formal operations:* Capable of abstract thought Can manipulate more than two categories of data at the same time Can think about the way others think	*Conventional to postconventional:* Able to make decisions based on their own set of internal moral values Questions the status quo and established rules

MILESTONES DURING THE FIRST YEAR

3 Months

- Raises head and chest when prone and can bring hands to mouth
- Follows a moving object with eyes
- Smiles at the sound of caregiver's voice, and smiles socially
- Begins to babble

7 Months

- Rolls from front to back and back to front
- Begins to sit with, then later without, support
- Transfers object from one hand to another and finds partially hidden objects
- Assumes hands-and-knees position
- Uses voice to express pleasure

12 Months

- Gets to sitting position without assistance
- Crawls forward on belly using arms and legs to push
- Responds to own name, will say "dada" and "mama," and tries to imitate words
- Uses pincer grasp

PHYSICAL CHANGES ASSOCIATED WITH NORMAL AGING

Body System	Physical Change
Bones and joints	Bones become less dense, are weaker, and are more likely to break.
	Bone density decreases after menopause in women due to estrogen loss.
Muscles and body fat	Amount of muscle tissue and muscle strength tends to decrease.
	Levels of growth hormone and testosterone decrease.
Eyes	Lens stiffens, making focusing on close objects harder.
	Lens becomes denser, making seeing in dim light harder.
	Lens yellows, changing the way colors are perceived.
	Pupils react more slowly to changes in light.
	Nerve cells decrease, impairing depth perception.
	The eyes produce less fluid, making them feel dry.
Ears	Exposure to loud noise over time damages the ear's ability to hear.
	Hearing high-pitched sounds becomes more difficult.
Mouth and nose	Taste buds decrease in number and sensitivity.
	Sweet and salt tastes decrease.
	Smell diminishes as the nerve endings in the nose deteriorate.

Skin	Becomes thinner, less elastic, drier, and finely wrinkled. The fat layer under the skin thins.
Brain and nervous system	The number of nerve cells in the brain decreases. New connections are made between the remaining nerve cells. Blood flow to the brain decreases.
Heart and blood vessels	Blood vessels become stiffer so blood pressure increases.
Lungs	The muscles used in breathing weaken. The number of alveoli and capillaries in the lungs decreases. The lungs become less elastic.
Digestive system	Food is emptied from the stomach more slowly. The stomach cannot hold as much food because it is less elastic. In the large intestine, materials move through more slowly. Liver cells decrease; less blood flows through the liver. Liver enzymes that help the body process drugs and other substances work less efficiently.
Kidneys and urinary tract	The number of kidney cells decreases. Less blood flows through kidneys and blood is filtered less efficiently. Kidneys may excrete too much water and too little salt. Dehydration becomes more likely.

Continued

PHYSICAL CHANGES ASSOCIATED WITH NORMAL AGING—cont'd

Body System	Physical Change
Reproductive organs	*Women:* Most effects are related to menopause, when the levels of female hormones (particularly estrogen) decrease, menstrual periods end permanently, and pregnancy is no longer possible. The ovaries and uterus shrink; the tissues of the vagina become thinner, drier, and less elastic. *Men:* Levels of testosterone decrease, resulting in fewer sperm and a decreased sex drive (libido). Erectile dysfunction (impotence) becomes more common as men age.
Endocrine system	Growth hormone levels decrease, leading to decreased muscle mass. Aldosterone levels decrease, making dehydration more likely. Insulin is less effective and less insulin may be produced, increasing the risk of type 2 diabetes.
Immune system	The cells of the immune system act more slowly. Cancer is more common among older people. Vaccines tend to be less protective. Pneumonia and influenza are more common. Allergy symptoms may become less severe.

From Porter RS, Kaplan JL (Eds): *Changes in the body,* 2010, Merck Manual Online, *www.merckmanuals.com/professional/index.html.*

HEALTH CONSIDERATIONS BY AGE GROUP[1]

Young Adulthood

Health risks: Cigarette smoking, alcohol or illicit drug use, sexual violence, accidents/injuries.

Health promotion: Diet, exercise, quit smoking.

Prevention screenings: Pap smears, breast self-examination, human papillomavirus (HPV), testicular self-examination, mental health screens.

Middle Adulthood

Health risks: Cancer, cardiovascular disease, diabetes, partner violence, accidents/injuries.

Health promotion: Continue young adult plus the following: decrease cholesterol, identify and treat high blood pressure, stress reduction, discuss low-dose aspirin with care, blood pressure checks, domestic violence.

Prevention screenings: Continue young adult plus the following: colonoscopy, prostate examination, mammogram, mental health screens.

Older Adulthood

Health risks: Arthritis, osteoporosis, chronic lung disease, hearing/vision changes, cognitive changes, disability, heart disease, cancer, cerebrovascular disease, respiratory disease, pneumonia, influenza, diabetes complications.

Health promotion: Vaccinations, smoking cessation.

Prevention screenings: Cancer screening, diabetes, lipid disorders, osteoporosis, hypertension, fall risk, elder abuse.

---

[1]Yoost BL, Crawford LR: *Fundamentals of nursing: Active learning for collaborative practice*, St. Louis, 2016, Mosby.

SAFE PRACTICE ALERTS!

- Avoid feeding toddlers foods that present choking hazards, such as hot dogs, hard candy, and fruit with pits.
- Ensure that hospital crib side rails are up and locked into position and the overhead rails are down and locked into position before leaving the bedside.
- The presence of viral infection and the use of aspirin in children are linked to Reye's syndrome, a potentially fatal toxic encephalopathy. Avoid use of aspirin and non–aspirin-containing salicylates during febrile illnesses in children.
- School-age children are often more cooperative with procedures if they are offered a simple explanation of what is happening and what they can expect to feel.
- Always ask patients about their use of alcohol, nicotine products, and recreational drugs such as marijuana, cocaine, crack, and heroin.
- Perform screening for domestic violence as part of the assessment of all patients, female or male, knowing that abuse occurs in homosexual and heterosexual relationships.
- Many older adults remain sexually active until late in life; nurses should include education and counseling on safe sex practices for the older adult.
- The changes caused by aging to the baroreceptors makes it vital for nurses to check postural blood pressures in the elderly to prevent postural hypotension and falls.
- Examine the feet of a patient with diabetes at every clinical encounter.

CHAPTER 16

Vital Signs

SITUATIONS THAT REQUIRE VITAL SIGN ASSESSMENT

- Establishing a baseline on admission to a health care agency.
- As part of a physical assessment.
- Routine monitoring during an inpatient stay.
- With any change in health status, especially complaints of chest pain and shortness of breath or feeling hot, faint, or dizzy.
- Before and after surgery or invasive procedures to establish baselines and monitor effects.
- Before and after administration of medications that affect cardiac, respiratory, or thermal regulation systems.
- Before and after interventions such as ambulation.
- Detecting improvement in patient condition.
- Validating readiness for discharge or transfer from a unit.
- Before and after a medication that affects cardiovascular and respiratory function.

VITAL SIGN RANGES ACROSS THE LIFE SPAN

Age	Temperature	Pulse per Minute	Respirations per Minute	SpO$_2$	Blood Pressure (mm Hg)	
					Systolic	Diastolic
Newborn	96°-99.5° F 35.5°-37.5° C	80-160	30-80	>95%	60-90	30-60
1-6 yr old	99.4°-99.7° F 37.4°-37.6° C	80-140	20-40	>95%	74-100	50-70
6-14 yr old	98°-98.6° F 36.6°-37° C	75-110	15-25	>95%	84-130	54-80
15 yr old	97°-99° F 36.1°-37.2° C	50-90	15-20	>95%	94-120	60-80
Adult	95.9°-99.5° F 35.5°-37.5° C	60-100	12-20	>95%	90-120	60-90
Older adult	95°-99° F 35°-37.2° C	60-100	15-20	>95%	90-120	60-90

TIME REQUIRED FOR READING THERMOMETERS

Time Required for Reading Glass Thermometer
Oral: 3 to 5 minutes
Axillary: 9 to 10 minutes
Rectal: 2 to 4 minutes

Time Required for Reading Disposable Thermometer
Hold the thermometer in place until the chemically impregnated dots change color (≈45 seconds).

Time Required for Reading Electronic Thermometer
Hold the thermometer in place until the light or auditory signal indicates a reading.

Time Required for Reading Tympanic Thermometer
Hold the thermometer in place until the reading is displayed (≈2 seconds).

Distance of Insertion for Rectal Thermometer
Child: 1 inch
Adult: 1½ inches

TEMPERATURE CONVERSION CALCULATION

To convert to Fahrenheit: $F = (C \times 9/5) + 32$
To convert to Celsius: $C = (F - 32) \times 5/9$
Axillary: Oral minus 1° F
Rectal: Oral plus 1° F

FACTORS AFFECTING TEMPERATURE

Age: Infants and elderly adults respond drastically to change in temperature.
Exercise: Increasing exercise will increase heat production and increase body temperature.
Hormones: Fluctuations in hormones can cause fluctuations in temperature.

Stress: Physical and emotional stress can increase body temperature.

Circadian rhythm: Lower temperatures in morning; higher in afternoon.

Hormones: Progesterone will raise temperature.

Emotions: Anxiety will raise temperature.

AVERAGE NORMAL ADULT TEMPERATURE RANGES

	Fahrenheit	Centigrade
Oral	96.8-99.68	36.0-37.6
Axillary	95.9-98.6	35.5-37.0
Rectal	93.92-100.04	34.4-37.8
Tympanic	96.08-99.32	35.6-37.4
Temporal	96.98-99.14	36.1-37.3

CLINICAL SIGNS OF FEVER

Onset: Increased heart rate, increased respirations, pallor, cool skin, cyanosis, chills, decreased sweating, and increased temperature.

Course: Flushed, warm skin; increased heart rate and respiration; increased thirst; mild dehydration; drowsiness; restlessness; decreased appetite; weakness.

Abatement: Flushed skin, decreased shivering, dehydration, diaphoresis.

FEVER PATTERNS

Fungal (infection): Rises slowly and stays high.

Intermittent: Spikes but falls to normal each day.

Persistent or sustained: Either remains elevated or low grade; often caused by tumors of the central nervous system.

Relapsing: Febrile for several days, alternating with normal temperatures; often caused by parasites or urinary tract infections.

Remittent: Spikes and falls but not to normal; often noted with abscesses, tuberculosis, or influenza viruses.

Septic (infection): Wide peak and nadir, often rigors and diaphoresis; often caused by gram-negative organisms.

THERMAL DISORDERS

Frostbite: Damage is caused to skin caused by extreme cold. At or below 0° C (32° F), blood vessels close to the skin constrict.
Treatment: Warm slowly.

Heatstroke: Temperature above 42.2° C or 108° F.
Treatment: Ice to groin and axilla.

Heat cramps: Spasms of muscles.
Treatment: Replace fluids; watch for chilling.

Hyperthermia: Any temperature above normal; severe hyperthermia is indicated by temperatures at or above 42.2° C or 108° F.
Treatment: Replace fluids, watch for chilling.

HYPOTHERMIA STAGES

Stage 1: Body temperature drops by 1° C to 2° C (1.8° F to 3.6° F). Shivering occurs. Unable to perform complex tasks with the hands. Blood vessels in the outer extremities contract. Breathing becomes quick and shallow. Goose bumps form to create an insulating layer of air around the body.
Treatment: Warm slowly.

Stage 2: Body temperature drops by 2° C to 4° C (3.6° F to 7.2° F). Shivering becomes violent. Muscle miscoordination becomes apparent. Mild confusion, although the victim may appear alert.

Victim becomes pale, and lips, ears, fingers, and toes may be blue.
Treatment: Warm slowly.

Stage 3: Body temperature drops below approximately 32° C or 90° F. Shivering may stop, and difficulty speaking, sluggish thinking, and amnesia appear; inability to use hands and stumbling are usually present. Skin becomes blue and puffy, muscle coordination very poor, walking nearly impossible, and the victim exhibits incoherent or irrational behavior. Pulse and respiration rates decrease, but ventricular tachycardia or atrial fibrillation can occur. Major organs fail.
Treatment: Warm slowly.

NORMAL PULSE RANGES WITH AVERAGES
Newborns: 80-(140)-160 beats per minute
Infant: 80-(120)-140 beats per minute
Child: 75-(100)-110 beats per minute
Adult
    Women: 60-(80)-100 beats per minute
    Men: 55-(75)-95 beats per minute

RHYTHM
Regular: Normal.
Regular or irregular: Usually regular but occasionally irregular.
Bigeminal: Skips every other beat (monitor needed for detection).
Pulsus paradoxus (PP) (also paradoxic pulse and paradoxical pulse): An exaggeration of the normal variation in the pulse during the inspiratory phase of respiration in which the pulse becomes weaker as one inhales and stronger as one exhales. It is a sign that is

indicative of several conditions, including cardiac tamponade and lung diseases (e.g., asthma, chronic obstructive pulmonary disease).

VOLUME AND AMPLITUDE OF PERIPHERAL PULSES

0 = Absent

1 + = Weak or thready, may be difficult to palpate

2 + = Normal, able to palpate with normal pressure

3 + = Bounding, may be able to see pulsation

FACTORS AFFECTING PULSE RATE

- **Age:** Pulse rate generally decreases from birth to adulthood, then increases in the elderly.
- **Gender:** Women generally have higher rates than do men.
- **Fever:** Pulse rate generally increases 7 to 10 beats for each degree of temperature elevation.
- **Pain:** Pain will increase the rate of a person's pulse.
- **Emotion:** Fear, anger, anxiety, and excitement increase the pulse rate.
- **Stress:** Being under stress will increase the pulse rate.
- **Digestion:** The increased metabolic rate during digestion will increase the pulse rate.
- **Medications:** Medications will both increase and decrease a pulse rate.
- **Hypovolemia:** Will increase the pulse rate to assist in volume replacement.
- **Hypoxia:** The pulse will increase to increase the oxygen-carrying abilities.
- **Blood pressure**: In general, heart rate and blood pressure have an inverse relationship. When the

blood pressure is low, there is an increase in pulse rate as the heart attempts to increase the output of blood from the heart (cardiac output).

- **Electrolyte balance:**
  - If the amount of sodium is too high in your body, the heart rate will increase.
  - If the potassium level is low, the heart cannot function properly and the heart rate will decrease.

PULSE SITES

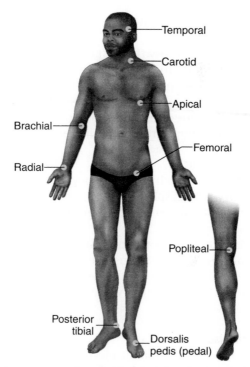

Pulse sites: temporal, carotid, apical, brachial, radial, femoral, popliteal, posterior tibial, pedal (dorsalis pedis).

HEART SOUNDS

S$_3$ (Ventricular Gallop)

Description: Low-frequency sound in early diastole.

Sounds like and location: Lub du bub S$_1$S$_3$S$_2$; cadence similar to "Ken-tuck-y."

Clinical significance: Results from increased atrial pressure leading to increased flow rates, as seen in congestive heart failure, which is the most common cause of an S$_3$. Often a normal physiologic finding in patients less than 30 years of age.

S$_4$

Description: Low-frequency sound in presystolic portion of diastole.

Sounds like and location: Belub dup S$_1$S$_4$S$_2$; cadence similar to "Tenn-ess-ee."

Clinical significance: Common in patients with stiffened left ventricles, resulting from conditions such as hypertension, aortic stenosis, and ischemic or hypertrophic cardiomyopathy.

Aortic Ejection Click

Description: Loud high-frequency sound, does not vary with respiration, most common early systolic sound; results from abrupt halting of semilunar valves.

Sounds like and location: Best heard at apex.

Clinical significance: Causes associated with aortic valve that has decreased mobility: that is, aortic stenosis, bicuspid aortic valves, and dilated aortic root.

Pulmonic Ejection Click

Description: Early systolic ejection sound with associated murmur. Often diminishes with inspiration.

Sounds like and location: Sternal edge second or third intercostal space.

Clinical significance: Causes associated with pulmonic valve: pulmonic stenosis, pulmonary hypertension, and dilated pulmonary trunk.

Opening Snap (OS)

Description: Early diastolic sound associated with mitral stenosis; often diminishes with inspiration and is best heard with patient in the left lateral position.

Sounds like and location: Between apex and left lower sternal border. Sounds like: RUP bu Dup rrrrrrRup Bu Dup; correlating to S_1, S_2, OS, murmur of mitral stenosis.

Clinical significance: Indicates the murmur is due to mitral stenosis.

Prosthetic Valves: Mitral Valve

Description: Mechanical or allograft.

Sounds like and location: Opening sound similar to opening snap and the closing sound coincides with S_1.

Clinical significance: Presence of a prosthetic mitral valve.

Prosthetic Valves: Aortic Valve

Description: Mechanical or allograft.

Sounds like and location: Opening sound similar to ejection click and the closing sound coincides with S_2.

Clinical significance: Presence of a prosthetic aortic valve.

Pericardial Friction Rubs

Description: Can be three-component rub that is a systolic sound between S_1 and S_2 or two-component rub in early diastole and at end diastole.

Sounds like and location: Over pericardium, often loudest at base of heart, rub often transient. Tends to be louder during inspiration. Sounds like scratching, grating, or squeaking. *Note:* Many patients with a pericardial friction rub also have tachycardia.

Clinical significance: Injury (shearing force) or inflammatory response to infection causes leakage or extra fluid into pericardium.

NORMAL RESPIRATION RANGES

Newborn and infant: 30 to 80 respirations per minute

Child: 24 to 40 respirations per minute

Adolescent: 15 to 25 respirations per minute

Adult: 12 to 20 respirations per minute

Older adult: 15 to 20 respirations per minute

RESPIRATORY ASSESSMENT

Depth: Deep or shallow

Rhythm: Even or uneven

Effort: Ease, quiet, or with great effort

Expansion: Symmetric or asymmetric

Cough: Productive, nonproductive, or absent

Auscultation: Clear, adventitious; crackles, wheezes; diminished, absent, no sounds

ABNORMAL PATTERNS OF BREATHING

Agonal respiration: Characterized by shallow, slow, irregular inspirations followed by irregular pauses. They may also be characterized as gasping or labored breathing accompanied by strange vocalizations. The cause is cerebral ischemia because of extreme hypoxia or even anoxia.

Apnea: Characterized by the cessation of respiration lasting for several seconds. Caused by respiratory distress syndrome, bronchopulmonary dysplasia, early cessation of theophylline or aminophylline, convulsions, intracranial or subdural hemorrhage, or cerebral edema.

Apneustic respiration: Characterized by deep, gasping inspiration with a pause at full inspiration followed by a brief, insufficient release. Caused by damage to the pons or upper medulla from strokes or trauma.

Ataxic respiration: Irregularity of breathing with irregular pauses and increasing periods of apnea. Caused by damage to the medulla oblongata because of strokes or trauma.

Cheyne-Stokes respiration: Rhythmic breathing with gradually increasing and decreasing tidal volume. Caused by the failure of the respiratory center.

Biot respiration or cluster respirations: Characterized by groups of quick, shallow inspirations followed by regular or irregular periods of apnea. Caused by damage to the medulla oblongata.

Bradypnea: Breathing rate is abnormally slow (<10 respirations per minute). Caused by depression of respiratory center by increased intracranial pressure, brain damage, or medications.

Hyperventilation: Overexpansion of the lungs characterized by rapid and deep breaths. May be caused by exercise, fear, anxiety, diabetic ketoacidosis, aspirin overdose.

Hypoventilation: Underexpansion of the lungs characterized by shallow slow respirations. May be caused by drug overdose or head injury.

Kussmaul breathing: Characterized by deep, regular breathing with a rate of fast, normal, or slow. Caused by metabolic acidosis, diabetic acidosis, and coma.

Sleep apnea: Characterized by temporary cessation of respiration. Caused by enlarged tonsils or adenoids, extreme obesity, or obstruction of the nasal airway.

Tachypnea: Breathing rate is increased (>24 respirations per minute), with quick, shallow breaths. Caused by fever, exercise, anxiety, respiratory disorders.

ADVENTITIOUS BREATH SOUNDS

Crackles: Most often in the lung bases and position-dependent lobes. Caused by the sudden opening of small airways and alveoli collapsed by fluid, exudate, or lack of aeration during expiration, pneumonia, atelectasis, cystic fibrosis, bronchitis, or pulmonary edema.

Pleural friction rub: Low-pitched, grating, or creaking sound. Can be described as the sound made by treading on fresh snow. Present over anterior lateral thorax, midline to axillae. Present during inspiration or expiration and is not cleared by cough. Occurs when inflamed pleural surfaces rub together during respiration.

Rhonchi: Low pitched, snore-like sounds heard either during inspiration or expiration, usually clear with cough. Continuous sounds, mainly heard over trachea and bronchi. Almost always caused by increased secretions in large airways.

Stridor: Intense, high-pitched, and continuous. Heard during inspiration, often heard without the aid of a stethoscope. Heard over trachea and large airways. Most often caused by epiglottitis, a foreign body lodged in the airway, or a laryngeal tumor.

Wheezing: High-pitched, whistling sound, heard continuously during inspiration or expiration; most obvious and loudest during exhalation.

Can be present in all lung fields. Most often caused by asthma, foreign objects, bronchiectasis, emphysema, pneumonia, heart failure, or gastroesophageal reflux.

NORMAL BLOOD PRESSURE AVERAGES (SYSTOLIC/DIASTOLIC)
Newborn: 60 to 90/30 to 60 mm Hg
Infant: 74 to 100/50 to 70 mm Hg
Child: 84 to 130/54 to 80 mm Hg
Adolescent: 94 to 120/60 to 80 mm Hg
Adult: 90 to 120/60 to 90 mm Hg
Older adult: 90 to 120/60 to 90 mm Hg

HYPERTENSION

Prehypertension	120-139 mm Hg	or	80-89 mm Hg
Stage 1 hypertension	140-159 mm Hg	or	90-99 mm Hg
Stage 2 hypertension	>160 mm Hg	or	>100 mm Hg

ORTHOSTATIC OR POSTURAL CHANGES
Take blood pressure and pulse with patient lying down. Then have patient sit or stand for 1 minute. Retake blood pressure and pulse. Record both sets of numbers. If patient is orthostatic, pressure will decrease (20 to 30 mm Hg) and pulse will increase (5 to 25 beats per minute) when sitting or standing. Record and report any orthostasis.

KOROTKOFF SOUNDS
Sounds of blood pressure:
Phase I: Systole (sharp thud)
Phase II: Systole (swishing sound)
Phase III: Systole (low thud or knocking)
Phase IV: Diastole (begins fading)
Phase V: Diastole (silence)

CARDIAC TERMINOLOGY
Blood volume: Amount of blood in the system.
Decreased blood volume: Equals decreased pressure, meaning increased need for fluids.
Increased blood volume: Equals increased pressure, meaning need for fewer fluids.
Cardiac output: Stroke volume multiplied by heart rate.
Diastole: Ventricular relaxation.
Pulse pressure: Systole minus diastole (normal range is 25 to 50).
Systole: Ventricular contraction.
Viscosity: Thickness of the blood.
Increased viscosity: Equals increased pressure, meaning more work on the heart.

BLOOD PRESSURE CUFF
Cuff should be 20% wider than the diameter of the limb.

Creating a False High Reading
- Having a cuff that is too narrow
- Having a cuff that is too loose
- Deflating the cuff too slowly
- Having the arm below the heart
- Having the arm unsupported
- Assessing blood pressure too soon after patient smoking or exercise

- Releasing the pressure valve too slowly
- Reinflating the bladder before it has completely deflated

Creating a False Low Reading
- Having a cuff that is too wide
- Having a cuff that is too tight
- Deflating the cuff too quickly
- Having the arm above the heart
- Hearing deficit of assessing person
- Ear tips of stethoscope placed incorrectly
- Breaks or kinks in cuff tubing
- Not placing stethoscope bell directly over artery

Creating a False Diastolic Reading
- Deflating the cuff too slowly
- Having a stethoscope that fits poorly in the examiner's ears
- Inflating the cuff too slowly

Creating a False Systolic Reading
- Deflating the cuff too quickly

PAIN: THE FIFTH VITAL SIGN
The words used by the patient to describe pain, such as *pressure, stabbing, sharp, tingling, dull, heavy,* or *cold.* It is important to use and understand the patient's language concerning pain and to believe the patient who reports pain.

PAIN ASSESSMENT[1]
Onset: Note when the pain first began, including the date and time.

----

[1]Adapted from McCaffery M, Beebe A: *Pain clinical manual for nursing practice,* ed 2, St. Louis 1999, Mosby.

Duration: How long does the pain last (persistent, minutes to hours, comes and goes, seconds)? Does the pain occur at the same time each day?

Location: In what area of the body does the pain begin? It may be helpful to have the patient point to the exact area if possible. *Note:* A patient may say the pain is in the stomach but may point over the lower abdominal area. Also ask if the pain radiates, moves, or goes to a different area of the body. Have the patient point to these areas as well.

Severity: How bad is the pain? Or have the patient rate the pain. Have a rating scale ready to use and explain your scale. Use the same scale in subsequent assessments. *Examples:* A 0 to 10 scale with 0 being no pain and 10 being the worst pain or a color scale with blue being no pain and red being the worst pain.

Precipitating factors: What was the patient doing before the pain began (exercise, bending over, work)?

Aggravating factors: What makes the pain worse?

Alleviating factors: What makes the pain get better or go away (pain medications, relaxation, rest, music)?

Associated factors: Nausea or vomiting, anger or agitation, depression or drowsiness, fatigue or sleeplessness.

Observed behaviors: Agitation or restlessness, bracing or fidgeting, rubbing or guarding, not eating or sleeping.

Vocalizations: Crying or moaning, gasping or groaning, sighing or noisy breathing.

Facial expressions: Grimacing or clenched teeth, wincing or furrowed brow, sadness or eyes closed, frightened or tightened lips.

PAIN RATING SCALES

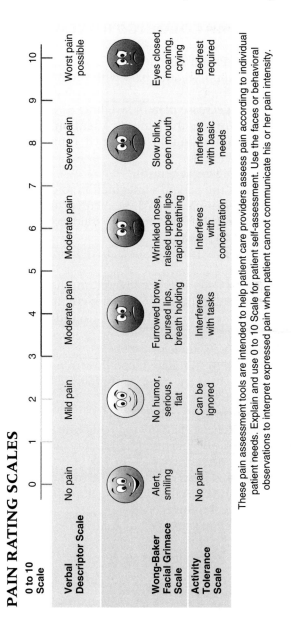

0 to 10 Scale	0	1	2	3	4	5	6	7	8	9	10
Verbal Descriptor Scale	No pain		Mild pain		Moderate pain		Moderate pain		Severe pain		Worst pain possible
Wong-Baker Facial Grimace Scale	Alert, smiling		No humor, serious, flat		Furrowed brow, pursed lips, breath holding		Wrinkled nose, raised upper lips, rapid breathing		Slow blink, open mouth		Eyes closed, moaning, crying
Activity Tolerance Scale	No pain		Can be ignored		Interferes with tasks		Interferes with concentration		Interferes with basic needs		Bedrest required

These pain assessment tools are intended to help patient care providers assess pain according to individual patient needs. Explain and use 0 to 10 Scale for patient self-assessment. Use the faces or behavioral observations to interpret expressed pain when patient cannot communicate his or her pain intensity.

NONPHARMACOLOGIC TREATMENT OF PAIN

Biofeedback: Patients can learn to control muscle tension to reduce pain with the use of biofeedback units.

Cold: Used to decrease pain or swelling.

Distraction: Turning the patient's attention to something other than the pain, such as music, visitors, or scenery.

Heat: Used to decrease tension.

Imagery: Uses the patient's imagination to create pleasant mental pictures. These pictures are a form of distraction. This activity is said to be a form of self-hypnosis.

Menthol: Used to increase blood circulation to painful areas.

Nerve blocks: Used to block severe, unrelieved pain. A local anesthetic, sometimes combined with cortisone, is injected into or around a nerve.

Positioning: See Chapter 24.

Pressure: Used to stimulate blood flow to painful areas. Apply firm but not excess pressure for 10 to 60 seconds.

Range of motion: See Chapter 24.

Relaxation: Relieves pain by reducing muscle tension. Music or relaxation tapes may be helpful.

Transcutaneous electrical nerve stimulation (TENS): A mild electric current is thought to interrupt pain impulses.

Vibration: Used to simulate blood flow to painful areas.

CHRONIC NONMALIGNANT PAIN: NURSING CARE GUIDELINES[2]

- Do not argue with the patient about whether he or she is in pain.
- Do not refer to the patient as a narcotics addict.
- Do not tell the patient that he or she will become an addict if he or she continues to receive narcotics.
- Do not use a placebo to try to determine if the patient has "real" pain.
- Be alert to any changes in the patient's pain condition or pain regimen.
- Recognize the differences between acute and chronic pain.
- Avoid sudden withdrawal of narcotics or sedatives from a patient with chronic pain.
- When analgesics are required, give them orally if possible. (The effects of oral analgesics will generally last longer than intravenous or intramuscular medications.) Review analgesics being used for relief of chronic versus acute pain.
- Offer pain relief alternatives.
- Review the patient's support systems and suggest additional ones if appropriate.
- Help those living with the patient to understand the patient's pain management routine.
- Assess the patient for depression, anxiety, and stress.

---

[2]Adapted from McCaffery M, Beebe A: *Pain clinical manual for nursing practice,* ed 2, St. Louis 1999, Mosby.

CRANIAL NERVES: FUNCTION AND ASSESSMENT

Number	Name	Type	Function	Method of Assessment
I	Olfactory	Sensory	Smell	Identify odors
II	Optic	Sensory	Vision	Snellen chart
III	Oculomotor	Motor	Vision	Pupil reaction
IV	Trochlear	Motor	Vision	Vertical vision
		Sensory	Cornea	Blink reflex
V	Trigeminal	Motor	Chewing	Clench teeth
VI	Abducens	Motor	Vision	Lateral vision
VII	Facial	Sensory	Taste	Identify tastes
		Motor	Expression	Smile or frown

VIII	Acoustic	Sensory	Equilibrium	Weber and Rinne tests
IX	Glossopharyngeal	Sensory	Taste	Identify tastes
		Motor	Swallowing	Gag reflex
X	Vagus	Sensory	Pharynx	Identify tastes
		Motor	Vocal	Voice tones
XI	Accessory	Motor	Shoulders	Shrug shoulders
XII	Hypoglossal	Motor	Tongue	Protruding tongue

SAFE PRACTICE ALERTS!

- Sudden alterations in vital signs or abnormal values become a priority situation for the nurse. Assessments and emergency measures should be initiated as indicated by the patient status. The health care provider is notified of alterations in vital signs.

- A temperature taken by the rectal route can cause bleeding in persons with hemorrhoids.

- Never palpate both carotid arteries at the same time to avoid limiting blood flow to the brain and causing the patient to experience syncope (fainting).

- If the peripheral pulse is irregular, count an apical pulse for 1 full minute to ensure accurate measurement.

- In infants and children younger than 2 years of age, the pulse rate is obtained by auscultating an apical pulse.

- Signs of respiratory distress include the use of accessory muscles of the chest and neck or exaggerated effort to breath. Children and infants may exhibit nasal flaring or sternal retractions if they are having trouble breathing.

- Be sure to assess the intensity, quality, duration, and location of pain. Assumptions of pain location may delay treatment for new symptoms and problems.

CHAPTER 17

Ethnicity and Cultural Assessment

CULTURAL TERMINOLOGY

Culture: The learned or shared values and beliefs of a particular group that are generally transferred from one generation to another.

Ethnicity: The individual's identification with or membership in a particular racial, national, or cultural group.

Enculturation: The process whereby a culture is passed from generation to generation.

Stereotypes: Fixed ideas or generalizations, often unfavorable, about members of a group.

Prejudice: The process of devaluing an entire group because of assumed behavior.

Discrimination: Policies and practices that harm a group and its members.

Race: A socially accepted process that groups people by common descent, heredity, or physical characteristics.

LEININGER'S STEPS FOR DELIVERY OF CULTURALLY COMPETENT CARE

1. Gain knowledge of the individual or family culture being assessed from reliable literature and through transcultural nursing courses taught by qualified faculty.

2. Know your own cultural heritage, patterns and biases, and factors that may interfere with an effective assessment and understanding of the patient.

3. Use theory or theoretical perspectives to guide your assessment such as the holistic Culture Care Theory with use of the Sunrise Model and Enabler.

4. Know some common language phrases of the patient to obtain accurate information and work with qualified interpreters.

5. Show respect and a genuine interest in the informant and the culture while remaining an active listener, letting the informant tell his or her story, experiences, and ideas to you.

6. Be observant of the environmental context in which you assess the patient and document your assessment.

7. As the patient shares information, reflect on and check the meaning of the data with the patient.

8. Make the patient an active co-participant in the assessment to obtain credible and accurate data.

9. Identify and then recheck specific and general cultural care values, beliefs, and needs related to data for possible integrated, culturally congruent nursing care.

10. Use assessment findings in sensitive, knowing, creative, and meaningful ways with the patient so that beneficial and satisfying outcomes are forthcoming. Do follow-up with the patient or family to document goal outcomes.

CHAPTER 18

Spiritual Health

COMMON SPIRITUAL BELIEFS THAT AFFECT HEALTH CARE[1]

Buddhism: Meditation calms the mind and body

Confucianism and Taoism:

- Moxibustion (use of the mugwort herb to promote circulation through warmth)
- Cupping (external suction therapy to improve circulation; usually employed for pain, respiratory problems, or digestive problems)
- Gua-sha therapy (rubbing applied to oiled skin to reduce fever and pain)
- Meditation is important aspect of healing
- Inclusion of family in decision making

Hinduism:

- Fasting to remove toxins (hot or cold food and drink also help remove toxins)
- Yoga or meditative practices
- Preference for modesty and same-sex caregivers
- Astrology, which can be part of decision making
- Belief that pain and suffering are due to bad karma
- Dietary restrictions, vegetarianism

---

[1]From Yoost BL, Crawford LR: *Fundamentals of nursing: Active learning for collaborative practice*, St. Louis, 2016, Mosby.

Islam:
- Privacy for prayer
- Preference for modesty and same-sex caregivers
- Family involvement in decision making
- Imam (religious leader) sometimes involved in decision making
- Dietary restrictions (no pork) and no or limited alcohol

Judaism: There are many sects, with varying levels of observance; the most common are identified by their beliefs and practices: Orthodox, Conservative, and Reformed
- Rites and rituals include specific foods and holiday observance
- Sabbath is Friday night to Saturday night, which may affect the acceptance of treatment during this time
- A newborn son is circumcised on the eighth day of life, during a ritual called a bris
- Circumcision is not performed in the hospital

Native American:
- The shaman, or medicine man or woman, helps restore health balance
- Healing rituals include herbal medicines, dances, songs, prayers, and sweat lodge ceremonies

Sikhism:
- Daily bathing, scripture reading, shaving restriction, modesty, and wearing of a turban head covering

CHAPTER 19

Public Health, Community-Based, and Home Health Care

Definitions (p. 127)
Vulnerable Populations (p. 128)
Assessment Questions Related to Community Health (p. 129)

DEFINITIONS[1]

- **Public health nursing** examines the greater community as a whole—the city, county, state, nation, continent, world—and designs collaborative and interdisciplinary strategies to keep the population healthy by preventing or controlling disease and threats to human health.
- **Community-based nursing** focuses on interventions necessary to help individuals prevent illness and maintain or regain their health while living in a community.
- **Home health care nursing** promotes, maintains, or restores health at an optimal level of functioning and reduces the effects of disability and illness for individuals and their families.
- **Case management** is the coordination of client care, needed services, and needed supplies in the home setting.

---

[1]From Yoost BL, Crawford LR: *Fundamentals of nursing: Active learning for collaborative practice*, St. Louis, 2016, Mosby.

- **Hospice care** or **palliative care** goals are to relieve suffering, to be a support to the client and family before the end of life, and to provide grief support after the death of the client.

VULNERABLE POPULATIONS[2]
Persons who are at particular risk for compromised health as a result of lack of resources, beliefs, life experiences and circumstances, or dependency include the following:

- Refugees and immigrants
- Individuals having experienced a natural or human-caused disaster
- Military personnel and veterans
- Workers prone to chemical or radiation exposure
- Homeless persons or families
- Minority groups within a larger population, including persons of various cultural, racial, religious, age, and genders that may be denied equal services based on their differences from the general population
- Mentally ill and disabled individuals
- Substance abusers or those with severe chronic illness
- Emotionally, physically, or sexually abused or neglected individuals
- Age-related populations such as the very young, adolescents, or elderly
- International foreign travelers

---

[2]From Yoost BL, Crawford LR: *Fundamentals of nursing: Active learning for collaborative practice,* St. Louis, 2016, Mosby.

ASSESSMENT QUESTIONS RELATED TO COMMUNITY HEALTH[3]

- What is the history of the community?
- Where have individuals worked historically and where do they work now?
- What sources of information exist to help in identifying key data?
- What are the environmental and sanitation services that protect the water supply, inspect restaurants, and license day care facilities?
- Where and what health promotion and educational services exist? Are there school nurses in each building?
- Are there public health clinics and health fairs?
- What preventive services are available, where, and to what populations?
- Are target populations able to access these services where they are being held?
- What matters to individuals within the community?
- Who are the stakeholders in the community and about what are they concerned?

[3]From Yoost BL, Crawford LR: *Fundamentals of nursing: Active learning for collaborative practice,* St. Louis, 2016, Mosby.

CHAPTER 20

Human Sexuality

SEXUAL HEALTH CHARACTERISTICS ACROSS THE LIFE SPAN

Infancy: Birth to 12 months
- **Characteristics:** Begins gender identification and body exploration.
- **Nursing implications:** Sexual self-manipulation is normal. Teach parents that this is normal at this stage.

Toddler: 1 to 3 years
- **Characteristics:** Continues with development of gender identification. Able to identify own gender.
- **Nursing implications**: Needs interaction with both male and female adults. Self-exploration and manipulation still normal.

Preschool: 3 to 5 years
- **Characteristics:** Increased self-awareness and begins asking questions about sex. Can identify body parts and name them. Exploration of own body parts and those of playmates are not uncommon.

- **Nursing implications:** Need to provide simple and direct answers to sex questions. Do not respond negatively to child's self-exploration. Best to identify body parts with appropriate names. Teach parents these guidelines.

School age: 6 to 12 years

- **Characteristics:** Engages in same-sex friendships. Has questions about physical and emotional aspects of sex. May begin development of primary and secondary sexual characteristics. Increased modesty noted. Strong identification with same-sex parent.
- **Nursing implications:** Answer sex-related questions honestly. Provide written information to assist with understanding. Discuss topics of sex, menses, and reproduction by 10 years. Respect modesty. Teach parents these guidelines.

Adolescence: 13 to 18 years

- **Characteristics:** Value system establishment. Development of primary and secondary sexual characteristics. Opposite-sex relationship development. Risk for pregnancy, sexually transmitted diseases (STDs), sexual abuse. Masturbation, homosexual relationships may be explored.
- **Nursing implications:** Recognize importance of peer group influences. Relationship with opposite sex sets stage for future. Teach pregnancy and STD information.

Young adult: 18 to 40 years

- **Characteristics:** Active sex life possible and establishment of values and lifestyle. Sharing of household and finances along with family planning and infertility. Homosexual identity established.

- **Nursing implications:** Provide information on pregnancy prevention, STDs. Need for open communication to work through issues of being a couple.

Middle adult: 41 to 65 years

- **Characteristics:** Reduced male and female hormone influences. Perimenopause/menopause. Quality versus quantity of sexual activity is now important.
- **Nursing implications:** Role adjustment in response to physiologic changes.

Older adult: 65 years and older

- **Characteristics:** Continued interest in sex; reduced sexual intercourse frequency. Female: Reduced vaginal secretions and breast atrophy. Male: Reduced sperm production and need for more time for erection and ejaculation.
- **Nursing implications:** Recognize continued interest in sex. Teach adaptation techniques to deal with any physical limitations that may interfere with sexual satisfaction.

SEXUAL HEALTH ASSESSMENT QUESTIONS[1]

- How do you feel about the sexual aspect of your life?
- Have you noticed any changes in the way you see yourself (as a man, woman, husband, wife, partner)?
- How has your (illness, surgery, medications) affected your sex life?
- Are you active sexually?
- Do you have problems or concerns as to your sexual (abilities, performance, satisfaction)?

---

[1]From Yoost BL, Crawford LR: *Fundamentals of nursing: Active learning for collaborative practice*, St. Louis, 2016, Mosby.

- How many sexual partners have you had in your lifetime?
- What are or have been your sexual practices?
- Do you feel safe in your environment?

CONTRACEPTION OPTIONS[2]
Barrier Methods
- **Diaphragm or cervical cap:** Placed inside the vagina to cover the cervix, before sexual intercourse with spermicide to block sperm. The diaphragm is shaped like a shallow cup. The cervical cap is a thimble-shaped cup.
- **Male condom:** Worn by the man to keep sperm from getting into a woman's body. Latex condoms, the most common type, help prevent pregnancy, as well as the transmission of HIV and other STDs, as do the newer synthetic condoms.
- **Female condom:** Worn by the woman to keep sperm from getting into her body. It is packaged with a lubricant. It can be inserted up to 8 hours before sexual intercourse. Also may help prevent the transmission of STDs.
- **Spermicides:** Products work by killing sperm. They are placed in the vagina no more than 1 hour before intercourse. Left in place for at least 6 to 8 hours after intercourse. Can use a spermicide in addition to a male condom, diaphragm, or cervical cap.

Hormonal Methods
- **Implant:** Single, thin rod that is inserted under the skin of a women's upper arm. The rod contains a progestin that is released into the body over 3 years.

---

[2]From Centers for Disease Control and Prevention (CDC): 24/7 Saving lives: Protecting people, *www.cdc.gov/reproductivehealth/ UnintendedPregnancy/Contraception.htm*.

- **Combined oral contraceptives:** Called "the pill," combined oral contraceptives contain the hormones estrogen and progestin. A pill is taken at the same time each day.
- **Progestin-only pill:** It may be a good option for women who cannot take estrogen.
- **Patch:** It releases the hormone progestin. Worn for 3 weeks, then not worn during the fourth week. Not worn so women can have a menstrual period.
- **Hormonal vaginal contraceptive ring:** Releases progestin and estrogen. Placed inside the vagina. Worn for 3 weeks, then removed for the week when the woman has her period, and then replaced with a new ring.
- **Emergency contraception:** Used after no birth control was used during sex or if the birth control method failed (e.g., broken condom).

Intrauterine Contraception
- **Copper T intrauterine device (IUD):** A small device that is shaped in the form of a "T." Placed inside the uterus. It can stay in the uterus for up to 10 years.
- **Levonorgestrel intrauterine system (LNG-IUD):** A small T-shaped device like the copper T IUD. Placed inside the uterus. It releases a small amount of progestin each day to keep patient from getting pregnant. The LNG-IUD stays in the uterus for up to 5 years.

Surgical Contraception
- **Female sterilization (tubal ligation or "tying tubes"):** The fallopian tubes are tied (or closed) so that sperm and eggs cannot meet for fertilization.

- **Transcervical sterilization:** A thin tube is used to thread a tiny device into each fallopian tube. It irritates the fallopian tubes and causes scar tissue to grow and permanently plug the tubes.
- **Male sterilization (vasectomy):** This operation is done to keep a man's sperm from reaching his penis, so his ejaculate never has any sperm in it that can fertilize an egg.

POTENTIAL SIDE EFFECTS OF MEDICATIONS

- **Anticonvulsants (phenytoin [Dilantin, Tegretol]):** Sedating effect and decreased sexual desire and function.
- **Antidepressants (tricyclics, monoamine oxidase inhibitors, lithium):** Male impotence and some reduction in testosterone levels.
- **Antihistamines:** Sedative effect can cause decreased desire and reduced female vaginal lubrication.
- **Antihypertensives (angiotensin-converting enzyme inhibitors, alpha and beta blockers, calcium channel blockers):** May decrease male and female desire and cause erectile dysfunction (ED).
- **Antipsychotics:** Reduce desire, ED, ejaculation dysfunction.
- **Antispasmodics:** Relax smooth muscle and may lead to male impotence.
- **Narcotics:** Increased dependence can result in increased sexual impairment; ED and ejaculation dysfunction is common; decreased male and female desire; decreased testosterone and semen production.
- **Alcohol (ethyl alcohol):** Moderate amount will reduce inhibition and may improve sexual function. Increased consumption leads to reduced

sexual function. Chronic alcoholism results in male impotence, permanent dysfunction, and sterility; in females, reduced desire and orgasmic dysfunction are possible.

- **Marijuana:** Initially may note reduced inhibitions and increased sexual function; with chronic use, male and female desire is decreased and male impotence may occur.

TERMS RELATED TO GENDER IDENTITY

- **Gender roles** are the outward behaviors of a person as a male or female and the perception of what are gender-appropriate actions.
- **Sexual orientation** is the attraction to one's own sex, the opposite sex, or both sexes when choosing a sexual partner.
- **Heterosexual** is defined as a person who has sexual interest in or sexual intercourse exclusively with partners of the opposite sex.
- **Homosexual** is defined as a person who has sexual interest in or sexual intercourse exclusively with members of his or her own sex. *Gay* is a term most often associated with male homosexuality, whereas *lesbian* refers exclusively to female homosexuality.
- **Bisexual** is an individual who is sexually active with others of either sex.
- **Transgendered** refers to having a gender identity or gender perception different from one's phenotypic gender.
- **Transvestite** is one who has the desire to dress in the clothes and be accepted as a member of the opposite sex.
- **Transsexual** is a person who has an overwhelming desire to be of the opposite sex. The sexual anatomy is not consistent with the gender identity. Transsexuals may choose cross-dressing (dressing in the clothing of the other

sex) or seek to have their external sex organs changed by transsexual surgery.

COMMON SEXUALLY TRANSMITTED DISEASES[3]

Chlamydia

Symptoms: May be asymptomatic; flu-like symptoms; genital discharge in men or women accompanied by burning with urination.

Transmission: During vaginal, oral, or anal sex or during vaginal delivery.

Prevention: Abstinence; monogamous relationship with uninfected partner; consistent and correct use of latex male condoms; annual testing of all sexually active women age 25 or younger and older women with new or multiple sex partners and all pregnant women.

Gonorrhea

Symptoms: May be asymptomatic; genital discharge, burning, and pain.

Transmission: Contact with the mouth, penis, vagina, or anus.

Prevention: Abstinence; monogamous relationship with uninfected partner; consistent and correct use of latex male condoms.

Human Papillomavirus (HPV)

Symptoms: May be asymptomatic, especially in males; genital warts develop with some types of HPV that vary in size and shape; can lead to various forms of cancer in both men and women.

Transmission: Vaginal, oral, and anal sex or genital-to-genital contact.

---

[3]From Centers for Disease Control and Prevention, 2012, *www.cdc.gov/std/default.htm.*

Prevention: Vaccines for girls and women: Cervarix and Gardasil; vaccines for boys and men: Gardasil; condom use may lower risk.

Syphilis

Symptoms: Three stages: beginning with sores, advancing to a rash and mucous membrane lesions and ending with a latent, late stage affecting the central nervous system and may lead to blindness, paralysis, and psychosis.

Transmission: Direct contact with syphilis sore (chancre) during vaginal, oral, or anal sex.

Prevention: Avoid alcohol and drug use, which may lead to risky sexual behavior; engage in sexual activity with a long-term monogamous partner who is known to be uninfected; consistent and correct use of latex condoms covering infected areas can reduce risk.

Genital Herpes

Symptoms: Genital discomfort; sores that heal within 2 to 4 weeks.

Transmission: Contact with sores during an outbreak or with infected skin between periods of outbreak.

Prevention: Abstain from sexual intercourse when lesions or symptoms are present; use condoms to reduce risk.

SAFE PRACTICE ALERT!

- Strict use of standard precautions including hand washing and use of clean gloves is imperative when providing nursing care to patients with suspected or verified STIs.

Nursing Principles

For more in-depth information on nursing principles, consult the following:

Yoost BL, Crawford LR: *Fundamentals of nursing: Active learning for collaborative practice,* St. Louis, 2016, Mosby.

CHAPTER 21

Safety

LIFE SPAN SAFETY CONSIDERATIONS
Infant, Toddler, and Preschooler
Use only approved cribs and toys
Childproof home environment
Cut food in small pieces
Fence pool areas
Never leave unattended

School-age
Supervise swimming and water activities
Safety precautions for trampolines and other activities
Encourage the use of bicycle helmets

Adolescent
Monitor for depression, drug use, and alcohol use
Educate regarding safe sexual practices
Safety courses for motor vehicles
Limit exposure to violence from television, games, movies, Internet
Encourage the use of bicycle helmets

Adult
Workplace concerns such as stress, working overtime, or being out of work
Illicit substances and prescription drugs
Driving while impaired
Unprotected sex practices

Older Adult
Fall risks
Decreased senses and mobility
Medication safety precautions
Driving safety

POISON SAFETY
Poisoning involves the intentional or unintentional ingestion, inhalation, injection, or absorption through the skin of any substance that is harmful to the body.

The National Poison Control Center phone number in the United States is 1-800-222-1222.

Signs and symptoms of poisoning vary depending on the amount of toxin and route of absorption.

- Some poisons enlarge the pupils, whereas others shrink them.
- Some result in excessive drooling, whereas others dry the mouth and skin.
- Some speed the heart, whereas others slow the heart.
- Some increase the breathing rate, whereas others slow it.

- Some cause pain, whereas others are painless.
- Some cause hyperactivity, whereas others cause drowsiness.

Almost every possible sign or symptom of a poisoning can also be caused by a non–poison-related medical problem. A thorough assessment should be completed and medical attention should be advised.

FIRE SAFETY

Many health care facilities use the fire emergency response defined by the acronym **RACE:**

R: *Rescue* all patients in immediate danger and move them to safe areas.

A: *Alarm:* Activate the manual-pull station and/or fire *alarm* and have someone call 911.

C: *Contain* the fire by closing doors, confining the fire, and preventing the spread of smoke.

E: *Extinguish* the fire if possible after all patients are removed from the area.

Know the facility's fire drill and evacuation plan. Close windows and doors. Turn off oxygen supply. All extinguishers are labeled A, B, C, or D according to the types of fires they are meant to extinguish. Some extinguishers can be used for more than one type of fire and are labeled with more than one letter. The types of fires the letters correspond to are as follows:

A: Paper or wood

B: Liquid or gas

C: Electrical

D: Combustible metal

COMMON MEDICAL EMERGENCIES
Heart Attack

Signs and symptoms: Chest pain; shortness of breath, dyspnea, a squeezing, crushing, or heavy feeling in the chest, light-headedness; pain in the left arm or in the jaw, nausea.

Intervention: Calm the patient and turn on the call light. Begin oxygen at 2 L if nearby. Remain calm and stay with the patient until help arrives. Document symptoms and actions taken.

Cardiac Arrest
Remain calm and turn on the call light and activate the facility internal emergency system. Begin cardiopulmonary resuscitation (CPR) (follow standard guidelines) until more experienced staff arrives and takes over. Clear furniture from the room and ask family to move to waiting area. (Some facilities allow family to watch CPR activity.)

Pulmonary Embolism
Signs and symptoms: Chest pain, shortness of breath, dyspnea, cyanosis, and possible death.
Causes: Immobility, deep vein thrombosis.
Intervention: Calm patient and turn on the call light and activate the facility internal emergency system. Begin oxygen at 2 L if nearby. Remain calm and stay with the patient until help arrives. Document symptoms and actions taken.
Prevention: Elevate legs, use antiembolism stockings, dorsiflexion of foot, perform range-of-motion exercises, check Homans sign, perform coughing and deep breathing exercise, and administer low dosages of heparin as prescribed while patient is hospitalized. Do not massage lower legs.

Shock
Mild or early: Warm, flushed skin, changes in orientation, widening pulse pressure.
Moderate or mild: Cool, clammy, pale skin; hypotension; narrowing pulse pressure; sweating; pallor; rapid pulse; decrease in urinary output.

Severe or late: All of the symptoms of moderate or mild shock plus irregular pulse, oliguria, shallow, rapid breathing, obtunded, or comatose.

Causes: Hemorrhage, infection, or hypovolemia.

Intervention: Monitor vital signs, assess orientation, and keep the patient warm. Record all symptoms and vital signs.

SEIZURE TERMINOLOGY

Absence seizure: Previously called *petit mal.* This is a generalized seizure *without* shaking.

Aura: A warning of a seizure. The aura is an early part of the seizure itself.

Complex partial: The person is conscious but impaired.

Epilepsy: Recurrent unprovoked seizures.

Febrile seizures: Generally occur in infants and young children; they are most often generalized tonic-clonic seizures. They typically occur in children with a high fever, usually higher than 102° F.

Generalized tonic-clonic seizure: Previously called *grand mal. Tonic* means stiffening, and *clonic* means rhythmic shaking. There is abnormal electrical activity affecting the whole brain (thus the term *generalized*).

Partial seizure: Sometimes confused with *petit mal.* Only a part of the brain is affected.

Postictal state: The period after a generalized or partial seizure during which the person usually feels sleepy or confused.

Seizure: Abnormal electrical activity in the brain.

Simple partial: The patient remains alert and is behaving appropriately.

Status epilepticus (SE): A state of continuous or frequently reoccurring seizures lasting 30 minutes or more.

CARE OF THE PATIENT WITH SEIZURES

Equipment and Procedures

Bed should be in the lowest position.

Side rails should be *up* and padded.

Oxygen and suction equipment should be nearby.

Indicate "seizure precautions" on plan of care.

Note if patient has an aura before seizures.

Use digital thermometers, NOT glass thermometers.

Patients should shower rather than use a tub.

Always transport the patient with portable oxygen.

Patients with frequent generalized atonic seizures should wear helmets.

During the Seizure

Call for help and do NOT try to restrain the person.

STAY WITH THE PERSON and time the seizure.

Help the person to lie down. Place something soft under the head.

Turn the person on his or her side if possible.

Remove glasses and loosen tight clothing.

Do NOT place anything between the teeth.

Do NOT attempt to remove dentures.

Monitor the duration of the seizure and the type of movement.

After the Seizure

Turn the person to one side to allow saliva to drain; suction if needed.

Perform vital signs and neurologic checks as needed.

Do NOT offer food or drink until the person is fully awake.

Reorient the person.

Notify physician *unless* the person is being monitored specifically for seizures.

Notify physician *immediately* if seizure occurs without regaining consciousness or if an injury occurs.

Record all observations.

Document the time and length of the seizure and if there was an aura.

Document the sequence of behaviors during the seizures (e.g., eye movement).

Document an injury and what was done about it.

Note what happened with the person just after the seizure (did he or she reorient?).

SPECIAL PATIENT SITUATIONS

Hospitalized patients with the following problems may require additional safety measures:

Alcohol Withdrawal

Signs and symptoms: Confusion, sweating, pallor, palpitations, hypotension, seizures, coma. Protocols may vary by facility. Withdrawal protocols may include seizure precautions, keeping the side rails up and padded, taking vital signs frequently (every 30 to 60 minutes or per hospital protocol), and close observation. Provide a safe environment. Perform neurologic, memory, and orientation checks. Document any withdrawal activity and actions taken.

Bleeding or Hemorrhage

Locate the source of the bleeding. Apply direct pressure with a clean drape. Call for assistance but stay with the patient. Assess for early signs of shock such as a change in sensorium and later signs of shock such as hypotension; pale skin; and a rapid, weak pulse.

Prevention: Closely supervise confused or heavily medicated patients and patients just returning from surgery. Make sure surgical dressings are secure. Encourage patients to call for assistance if bleeding begins. Document any bleeding and actions taken.

Choking

Follow standard abdominal thrust maneuver guidelines.

Prevention: Closely supervise confused and heavily medicated patients. Make sure patients are sitting up or are placed in high Fowler position when eating. Encourage the use of the call lights. Assess the patient's ability to chew and swallow. Order a diet appropriate to the patient's eating ability. Document any choking situations and actions taken.

The Confused Patient

Assess for the source of the confusion. Possible sources include age, medications, disease, and infection. Confused patients may be at risk for falls.

Drug Reactions

Assess for difficulty breathing, wheezing, tearing, palpitations, skin rash, pruritus, nausea or vomiting, rhinitis, diarrhea, and a change in mood or mental status. These are general drug reactions, not the side effects of specific drugs. Immediately report all drug reactions.

Prevention: Closely supervise confused and heavily medicated patients and patients who are taking medications for the first time. Encourage the use of the call lights if any of the signs of a drug reaction occur. Know your patient's drug allergies. Document all drug reactions and actions taken.

SYNCOPE AND COMMON CAUSES

Neurologic: Vertebrobasilar transient ischemic attacks, subclavian steal syndrome, hydrocephalus.

Metabolic: Hypoxia, hyperventilation, hypoglycemia.

Cardiac: Orthostatic hypotension, vasovagal reaction or syncope.

Vasomotor: Obstructive lesions, arrhythmias. Assess for dizziness, light-headedness, visual blurring or any visual or hearing changes, weakness, apprehension, nausea, sweating, blood pressure, and pulse.

Prevention or intervention: Stay with the patient. Help the patient sit or lower to the chair, bed, or floor. Protect the patient's head at all times. Call for help. Elevate the legs, assess vital signs, use ammonia (if needed), help the patient sit up slowly when he or she is ready, and document per organizational policy.

MORSE FALL SCALE ASSESSMENT

Risk Factor	Scale	Score
History of falls	Yes	25
	No	0
Secondary diagnosis	Yes	15
	No	0
Ambulatory aid	Furniture	30
	Crutches/cane/ walker	15
	None/bed rest/ wheelchair/nurse	0
IV/heparin lock	Yes	20
	No	0

Continued

Risk Factor	Scale	Score
Gait/transferring	Impaired	20
	Weak	10
	Normal/bed rest/ immobile	0
Mental status	Forgets limitations	15
	Oriented to own ability	0

To obtain the Morse Fall Score add the score from each category.

Morse Fall Score

High risk	45 and higher
Moderate risk	25-44
Low risk	0-24

FALL PREVENTION AT THE HOSPITAL[1]

- Frequently observe the patient.
- Place the patient in a room near the nurses' station.
- Use a low bed.
- Use a mattress or wheelchair seat with pressure alarms.
- Use side rails. (*Note:* Use of four side rails is considered a restraint.)
- Always return the bed to its lowest position.

---

[1]From Yoost BL, Crawford LR: *Fundamentals of nursing: Active learning for collaborative practice,* St. Louis, 2016, Mosby.

- Keep the call bell within reach of the patient.
  - Remind the patient about how to use the call bell.
  - Immediately answer the call bell if it is sounded.
- Keep the wheels of any wheeled device (bed, wheelchair) in the locked position.
- Leave lights on or off at night depending on the patient's cognitive status and personal preference.
- Keep personal items (tissues, water, urinals) within the patient's reach.
- Frequently orient and reorient the patient.
- If the patient is ambulatory, require the use of nonskid footwear.
- Clear any potential obstructions from the walking areas.
- Ensure that patient clothing fits properly; improper fit can cause tripping.

Fall Assessment Checklist

One or more of the following items can place a person at risk for falls:

- Agitated
- Cardiac disease
- Disoriented or confused
- Diuretic use
- Does not speak or understand English
- Electrolyte imbalance
- Hearing or visual loss
- History of falls
- Hypotensive
- Neurologic disease
- Older than 70 years of age
- On new medication
- Peripheral vascular disease
- Psychotropic drug use
- Recent cerebrovascular accident
- Recent myocardial infarction
- Uncontrolled diabetes
- Urinary frequency
- Uses cane or walker
- Weak

RESTRAINTS
When to use:
- To prevent injury
- To restrict movement
- To immobilize a body part
- To prevent harm to self or others

Restraints should be used only when all other methods of keeping a patient safe have been tried.

Know the organizational policy regarding the use of restraints.

Types of Restraints
Jackets or vests, belts, mittens, wrist or ankle, crib net, elbow

Guidelines
- Obtain physician's order and follow facility protocol.
- Explain purpose to patient; check circulation every 30 minutes.
- Release temporarily (once per hour).
- Provide range of motion.
- Document need and examination schedule.
- Report problems and tolerance; provide emotional support.
  Never secure restraints to the side rails or the nonstationary portion of the main frame of the bed.

Complications
- Skin breakdown (pad bony areas).
- Nerve damage (do not overtighten; release often).
- Circulatory impairment (check for problems often; provide range of motion).
- Death (from inadequate or improper use).

Prevention
- Keep the side rails up when you are not with the patient.

- Monitor vital signs and the patient's drug doses and levels.
- Monitor the patient's electrolytes and neurologic status.
- Reorient patient to place and time as needed.
- Place call light in easy reach.
- Attend closely to personal care needs.
- Encourage family, friends, and clergy to visit often.

HOW TO TIE A QUICK-RELEASE (POSEY) TIE

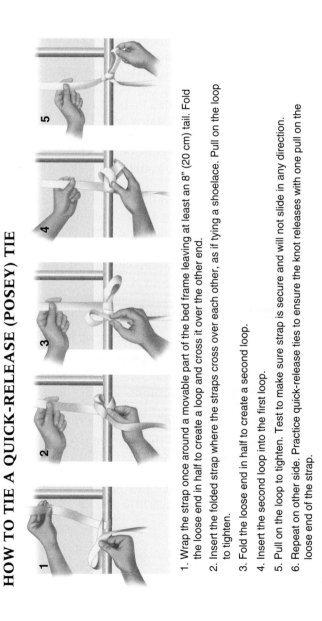

1. Wrap the strap once around a movable part of the bed frame leaving at least an 8" (20 cm) tail. Fold the loose end in half to create a loop and cross it over the other end.

2. Insert the folded strap where the straps cross over each other, as if tying a shoelace. Pull on the loop to tighten.

3. Fold the loose end in half to create a second loop.

4. Insert the second loop into the first loop.

5. Pull on the loop to tighten. Test to make sure strap is secure and will not slide in any direction.

6. Repeat on other side. Practice quick-release ties to ensure the knot releases with one pull on the loose end of the strap.

FALL PREVENTION AT HOME[2]

Health teaching for patients discharged to or residing in the home needs to include environmental interventions for fall prevention.

- Remove obstacles from walking paths (clutter, throw rugs, and cords).
- Ensure adequate lighting in areas such as bathrooms, halls, and stairways.
- Use nightlights in common areas such as hallways or in walkways to the bathroom.
- Keep assistive devices (canes and walkers) within reach.
- Repair loose or uneven floor/stairway surfaces.
- Install and maintain handrails and grab bars.
- Use devices such as long-handled grabbers rather than reaching or stooping.
- Keep frequently used items close by or within reach.
- If there are children in the house, are gates installed in doorways and at the top and bottom of stairs?

HOME SAFETY ASSESSMENT[3]

Health history and physical assessment should dictate specific safety questions, such as the following:

- **Activities of daily living:** Do you require assistance with any of the following: walking, toileting, bathing, dressing, grooming, eating, cooking, driving, shopping, or cleaning?
- **Medications:** Do you know how and when to take your medications? Do you know why

[2,3] From Yoost BL, Crawford LR: *Fundamentals of nursing: Active learning for collaborative practice*, St. Louis, 2016, Mosby.

you take them? Do you take your medications consistently? Have you been experiencing any side effects? If yes, describe them. Where are your medications stored? Are they out of reach of children, or do they have childproof caps? Are any medications expired?

- **Health issues:** Do you have any injuries or health issues that place you at risk for falling or for drowsiness? Have you ever had a seizure?
- **Safety issues:** Do you have any safety concerns? Do you have a history of falling? Do you have worries about what you would do in case of a fire? Are you stressed out or tired?
- **Chemicals:** How do you store your household chemicals? Are they out of reach of children and pets?
- **Carbon monoxide:** Do you have a carbon monoxide detector in your home?
- Do you have adequate outlets for all of your appliances and electronic devices? If there are children in the home, are all outlets in your home covered?
- Do you check for frays or loose wires on electrical cords, including those of electronic devices such as laptops and cell phones?
- Are your circuit breaker boxes in working order?
- Are household appliances, such as irons, hair dryers, and electric razors, used away from sources of water? Are the electrical outlets grounded?
- Do you have smoke detectors? A fire extinguisher? An evacuation plan in case of a fire?
- Do you smoke, or does anyone in your home smoke?
- **Needles:** Do you use hypodermic needles? How do you dispose of them?

- How do you heat your home? Is it adequate? Do you use space heaters?
- Do you have screens in your windows in the summer?
- Do you have air-conditioning? Fans?

SAFE PRACTICE ALERTS!

- Frequent checks of the patient under restraint are essential because injuries due to entrapment and death from strangulation or asphyxiation are most likely to result when the patient attempts to escape physical restraint.
- Never tie a restraint in a knot because the knot could prohibit quick exit in the event of an emergency requiring evacuation. Instead, use quick-release ties or mechanisms such as buckles. Restraints should never be tied to side rails because injuries could result with raising or lowering.

CHAPTER 22

Asepsis and Infection Control

TERMINOLOGY

Asepsis: Prevention of the transfer of microorganisms and pathogens.

Chain: Path of infection; the components of the infectious disease process.

Clean: Presence of few microorganisms or pathogens with no visible debris.

Colonization: Presence of a potentially infectious organism in or on a host but not causing disease.

Communicable: Ability of a microorganism to spread disease.

Contamination: Presence of an infectious agent on a surface.

Dirty: Presence of many microorganisms or pathogens; any soiled item.

Disease: Alteration of normal tissues, body processes, or functions.

Etiology: Cause of a disease.

Fungi: Single-cell organisms that are capable of causing infection.

Immunity: Resistance to a disease associated with the presence of antibodies.

Infection: Invasion of tissues by a disease-causing microorganism(s).

Medical asepsis: Measures that limit pathologic spread of microorganisms.

Nosocomial infection: A hospital-acquired infection (not present or incubating on admission).

Parasites: Organisms that live on or in other organisms.

Ports: How microorganisms exit and enter a system.

Reservoir: Storage place for organisms to grow.

Source: Point that initiates chain of infection.

Sterile: Absence of all microorganisms.

Surgical asepsis: Measures to keep pathogenic organisms at a minimum during surgery.

Transmission: Method by which microorganisms travel from one host to another.

Virulence: Ability of a microorganism to produce disease.

Vector: Carries a pathogen from one host to another.

STAGES OF INFECTION

Incubation: From initial contact with infectious material to onset of symptoms.

Prodrome: From nonspecific signs and symptoms to specific signs and symptoms (prodromal).

Illness: Presence of specific signs and symptoms.

Convalescence: During the recovery period as symptoms subside.

THE INFLAMMATORY PROCESS

Stage I

Constriction of blood vessels, dilatation of small vessels, increased vessel permeability, increased leukocytes, swelling, and pain. Leukocytes begin to engulf the infection.

Stage II

Exudation with fluids and dead cells.

Serous: Clear; part of the blood.

Purulent: Thick; pus with leukocytes.

Sanguineous: Bloody.

Stage III

Repair of tissues.

Regeneration: Same tissues.

Stroma: Connective tissues.

Parenchyma: Functional part.

Fibrous: Scar.

CHAIN OF INFECTION

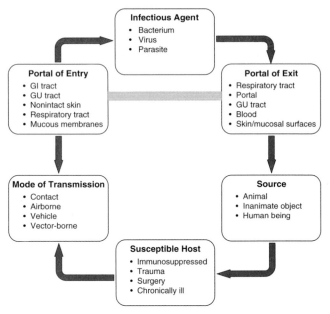

TYPES OF IMMUNITY

- **Cellular immunity:** Involves a defense by the white blood cells—T lymphocytes—in response to foreign microorganisms.
- **Humoral immunity:** A defense system that involves antibodies and white blood cells that are produced to fight antigens.
- **Innate immunity:** Protects the body against foreign antigens. The skin, cough reflex, mucus, enzymes on the skin and in tears, and acid in the gastrointestinal tract are all part of the body's innate immunity.

- **Active immunity:** Antibodies produced in the body after exposure, generally long-lasting.
  - Natural—produced from active infection such as chickenpox, mumps, measles.
  - Artificial—vaccine of antigens such as measles, mumps, rubella (MMR).
- **Passive immunity:** Antibodies produced outside of the body, generally short acting.
  - Natural—passed from mother to child through placenta or breast milk.
  - Artificial—antibodies introduced through injection of immune serum.

ANTIBODY FUNCTIONS
IgM: First to respond; activates the complement system; stimulates ingestion by macrophage; principal antibody of the blood.

IgG: Most prevalent antibody; major antibody of the tissues; produced after IgM; only antibody to cross placenta; antitoxin; antiviral.

IgA: Principal antibody of the GI tract; found in tears, saliva, sweat, breast milk; protects epithelial lining.

IgD: Only in minute concentrations; function unknown.

IgE: For allergic reactions.

INFECTION ASSESSMENT
- **Vital signs:** Often the first indication of an infection.
  Temperature, pulse, respirations, and blood pressure generally elevate.
  The lowering of blood pressure is a late sign of sepsis.
- **Nutrition status:** Proteins, vitamins, and water all deplete during an infection.

- **Risk assessment:** People at risk for infection are those with chronic disease, on chemotherapeutic agents, or with indwelling catheters and those who may be malnourished.
- **Laboratory and diagnostic tests:** Complete blood count (CBC), including a differential white blood cell (WBC) count.

  The normal WBC count for adults is 4500 to 10,500 cells/mm^3.

  A shift to the left with a higher percentage of neutrophils than normal indicates an infection.

  A culture and sensitivity of the blood, urine, stool, or wound drainage may be indicated.

TYPES OF PRECAUTIONS
Standard Precautions

- Prevents and controls the spread of microorganisms among patients and providers.
- Used during contact or potential contact with the following:
  - Blood and bodily fluids (except perspiration), secretions, and excretions (and *must* be used whether or not blood is visibly present).
  - Nonintact skin, mucous membranes.
  - Other potentially infectious material (OPIM).
- Use gloves routinely.
- If splashing is possible, use other personal protective equipment (PPE).
  - Eyewear, a mask, and a gown.
- Practice good hand hygiene. (See Indications for Hand Hygiene in Chapter 23.)
- Equipment must be cleaned or discarded after use.

- Follow special precautions when using needles (sharps):
  - Discard needles in sharps containers.
  - Use safety needles.
  - Needleless systems are preferred when their use is feasible.
  - Educate patients and staff regarding the procedure to be performed on the patient.

Transmission-Based Precaution Guidelines

- Standard Precautions apply to all patients.
- Personal protective equipment/supplies should be found on the isolation cart and are located per the organization policy.

Contact Precautions are used when a known or suspected contagious disease may be present.

- Transmission of a contagious disease may be through *direct transmission* (contact with the patient) or *indirect transmission* (contact with equipment or items in the patient's environment).
  - Examples of typical diseases/conditions:
    - Multidrug-resistant organisms (MDROs): vancomycin-resistant enterococci (VRE), methicillin-resistant *Staphylococcus aureus* (MRSA), *Clostridium difficile* (C. diff), respiratory syncytial virus (RSV), hepatitis A.
    - Scabies, herpes simplex virus (HSV).
    - Draining wounds in which secretions cannot be contained.

Airborne Precautions are used when known or suspected contagious diseases can be transmitted through small droplets or particles that can remain suspended in the air for prolonged periods of time.

- Precautions may include the following:
  - A negative-pressure room with a high-efficiency particulate air (HEPA) filtration system may be necessary.
  - A special N95 respirator mask is required: must be fit-tested.
- Typical diseases/pathogens include varicella or disseminated varicella zoster (chickenpox); rubeola (measles); and *Mycobacterium tuberculosis* (pulmonary or laryngeal tuberculosis [TB]).

Droplet Precautions are used when known or suspected contagious diseases can be transmitted through large droplets contained in the air.

- Droplets may be generated when an infected patient coughs, sneezes, or talks or during medical procedures such as suctioning, endotracheal intubation, cardiopulmonary resuscitation (CPR), or chest physiotherapy.
- Typical diseases include pharyngeal diphtheria, mumps, rubella, pertussis, streptococcal pharyngitis, scarlet fever, pneumonias (streptococcal, mycoplasmal, meningococcal), pneumonic plague, meningococcal sepsis, and influenza.

Protective Precautions are used to protect people from microorganisms in the environment secondary to immune issues.

- Protective precautions are taken because of immune issues related to disease conditions or treatment.
- A variety of protective precautions may be used.
  - A positive-pressure room with a HEPA filtration system may be required.

- A special respirator mask may be required: must be fit-tested.
- Meticulous hand washing is essential.
- Patient must be assessed carefully for signs and symptoms of infection.
- No live plants, fresh flowers, fresh raw fruit or vegetables, sushi, or blue cheese may be brought into the room because they may harbor bacteria and fungi.

- Typical conditions requiring protective precautions include allogeneic hematopoietic stem cell transplantation, chemotherapy, and certain disease conditions or when medications have caused immunosuppression (including leukemia, myelodysplastic syndrome, aplastic anemia, systemic lupus erythematosus [SLE], rheumatoid arthritis [RA], human immunodeficiency virus [HIV], severe sepsis, and others).

PREVENTION OF SPREAD OF RESISTANT PATHOGENS

- Wash hands and use alcohol-based hand sanitizers to reduce the spread of bacteria.
- Adhere to all organizational infection control policy and procedures.
- Use patient-specific equipment for patients when possible.
- Clean environmental surfaces regularly and when soiled.
- Use personal protective equipment (PPE) according to facility's infection control policy.
- Use antibiotics only when needed and complete each course of antibiotics as prescribed.

ANTIBIOTIC-RESISTANT PATHOGENS

Acinetobacter baumannii: Multidrug-resistant (MRAB)

Clostridium difficile: Clindamycin resistant;
fluoroquinolone-resistant ciprofloxacin (Cipro)
and levofloxacin (Levaquin)

Escherichia coli: 80% of the bacteria are resistant to
one or more drugs

Enterococcus: Vancomycin-resistant (VRE; see below)

Mycobacterium tuberculosis: Multidrug-resistant
(MDR-TB)

Salmonella: Resistant to nine different antibiotics

Staphylococcus aureus: Methicillin-resistant (MRSA;
see below); linezolid-resistant; vancomycin-
resistant (VRSA); community-acquired
(CA-MRSA)

Streptococcus pyogenes (group A strep):
Macrolide-resistant

Streptococcus pneumoniae: Penicillin-resistant

MRSA AND VRE

MRSA: Methicillin-resistant *Staphylococcus aureus*

VRE: Vancomycin-resistant *Enterococcus* organisms

Standard Precautions for MRSA

Masks: Necessary if patient's respiratory tract
is colonized or has an active infection; must
use when suctioning or when patient has a
productive cough.

Gowns: Necessary if in contact with secretions.

Gloves: Necessary for all contact with items that
may be contaminated.

Private room: If possible or with other patients
with MRSA and no other infections.

Standard Precautions for VRE

Masks: Necessary if contact with secretions is
likely.

Gowns: Necessary if contact with secretions is likely.

Gloves: Necessary for all contact with items that may be contaminated

Private room: If possible or with patients who have VRE and no other infections.

COMMON INFECTIOUS DISEASES

- Standard Precautions are required for all people with infectious diseases (see Types of Precautions, earlier in this chapter).
- Check state requirements for reporting infectious diseases.

AIDS/HIV

Transmission through blood and body fluids, sexual contact, sharing IV needles, contaminated blood, and from mother to fetus.

Considerations: Education regarding mode of transmission, avoidance of sexual contact with infected people, use of latex condoms, proper blood screening of all transfusable products, and proper handling of needles and other contaminated material.

Chickenpox/Herpes Zoster Virus (Varicella/Shingles)

Transmission through respiratory droplets or by direct contact with open lesions.

Considerations: Contact isolation, avoid direct contact with lesions, and administration of varicella zoster immune globulin. Caregivers should be chickenpox immune. The chickenpox vaccine is becoming more commonly used, and a single-dose shingles vaccine is recommended for people over 60 years. About 90% of unvaccinated people will catch chickenpox if exposed. Shingles and pneumococcal vaccines should not be given during the same medical visit.

Chlamydia

Transmission through sexual contact.

Considerations: Public education and use of latex condoms.

German Measles (Rubella)

Transmission through respiratory droplets.

Considerations: Education regarding vaccines and prenatal care, and avoidance of contact.

Gonorrhea

Transmission through vaginal secretions, semen, sexual contact.

Considerations: Public education regarding mode of transmission and use of latex condoms. Some strains are antibiotic resistant.

Hepatitis A and Hepatitis E

Transmission through direct contact with water, food, or feces.

Considerations: Hand hygiene before touching food, proper water and sewage treatment, reporting of cases, immunoglobulin vaccination when traveling to high-risk areas, proper disposal of contaminants. A combination vaccine for hepatitis A and B is now available.

Hepatitis B

Transmission through all fluids of an infected source. No treatment is available. Hepatitis B infection kills over 5000 Americans each year and is the leading cause of liver cirrhosis and liver cancer.

Considerations: Hepatitis B vaccination (three doses given over 6 months), public education, blood screening, use of gloves when

handling secretions, proper sterilization of
equipment, reporting of all known cases.

Hepatitis C
Transmission through contaminated blood, plasma,
and needles.
Considerations: See Hepatitis B.

Hepatitis D
Hepatitis D can develop only in individuals who
have active hepatitis B and in those who are
carriers of hepatitis D.

Measles (Red, Hard, Morbilli, Rubeola)
Transmission through airborne droplets or direct
contact with lesions; 20% of people experience
one or more complications.
Considerations: Public education about vaccine
and avoidance of contact with infected people.

Meningitis (Bacterial)
Transmission through airborne droplets or direct
contact.
Considerations: Public education, vaccination, and
early prophylaxis of exposed contacts.

Mononucleosis
Transmission through saliva.
Considerations: Public education and good
hygiene.

Mumps
Transmission through airborne droplets and saliva.
Considerations: Vaccination.

Pneumonia
Transmission through airborne droplets.

Considerations: Vaccination and good hygiene. Some some strains are antibiotic resistant.

Polio (Poliomyelitis)
Transmission through oral or fecal contact.
Considerations: Vaccination.

Salmonellosis
Transmission through ingestion of contaminated food.
Considerations: Proper cooking and storage of food and good hand hygiene before food preparation.

Syphilis
Transmission through sexual contact, direct contact with lesions, and blood transfusions.
Considerations: Public education regarding transmission, prenatal screening and prenatal follow-up, use of latex condoms, and blood screening.

Tetanus (Lockjaw)
Transmission through direct contact of wounds with infected soil or feces; 16% of cases are fatal.
Considerations: Public education regarding mode of transmission, vaccination.

Tuberculosis
Transmission through airborne droplets; bovine TB through unpasteurized milk.
Considerations: Public education and screening, improvement of overcrowded living conditions, and pasteurization of milk.

Typhoid Fever
Transmission through contaminated water, urine, or feces.

Considerations: Good hygiene, sanitary water, proper sewage care, and vaccinations.

Whooping Cough (Pertussis)

Transmission through airborne droplets and nasal discharge, with the number of cases increasing during the past several years.

Considerations: Vaccination, wearing of masks when near infected patients, reporting of all cases. Adults under age 65 who have never gotten the Tdap booster should receive it for the next scheduled tetanus booster.

INFLUENZA

- Symptoms include fever, headache, dry mouth, fatigue, sore throat, cough, and muscle aches.
- Up to 20% of Americans get the flu each year.
- Influenza in conjunction with pneumonia is the sixth leading cause of death in the United States among older adults.
- A person cannot catch influenza from a vaccine.
- Because influenza viruses can change from year to year, an annual influenza shot is needed each fall.
- The best time to receive an influenza vaccine is October through December.
- Influenza vaccine will not protect from other illnesses, such as colds, bronchitis, and the stomach influenza or gastritis.
- Vaccinations can prevent up to 50% of the 140,000 hospitalizations and 80% of the 300,000 deaths that occur each year.
- Influenza can worsen heart and lung diseases and diabetes.
- Influenza can lead to pneumonia.

COMPARISON: COLD, INFLUENZA, AND PNEUMONIA

Cold

Caused by a virus.

Symptoms include runny nose and congestion, sore throat, cough.

Recovery time is 1 to 2 weeks.

Treatment is often symptom support with no need for antibiotics.

Severity is less than the flu.

Influenza

Caused by a virus.

Symptoms include fever, body aches, extreme fatigue, headache, congestion, cough.

Recovery time is 1 to 2 weeks.

Treatment is often symptom support with no need for antibiotics.

Can be severe.

Pneumonia

Can be caused by a virus or bacteria.

Symptoms can include fever, cough, and difficulty breathing.

Recovery time is usually longer than that of the flu.

Treatment will often require antibiotics (if caused by a bacterium).

Often severe and may require hospitalization.

HOME CARE CONSIDERATIONS TO PREVENT INFECTION[1]

- Teach proper hand hygiene (before handling foods, before eating, after toileting, before and after required home care treatment, and

---

[1]From Yoost BL, Crawford LR: *Fundamentals of nursing: Active learning for collaborative practice*, St. Louis, 2016, Mosby.

after touching body substances such as wound drainage) and related hygienic measures for all family members.

- Instruct the patient and family not to share personal care items, such as toothbrushes, washcloths, and towels.
- Discuss the use of antimicrobial soaps and effective disinfectants.
- Instruct about cleaning reusable equipment and supplies: Use soap and water, and disinfect with a chlorine bleach solution.
- Teach the patient and family members the signs and symptoms of infection, how to avoid infections, and when to contact a health care provider.
- Remind the patient and family members to avoid coughing, sneezing, or breathing directly on others. Cover the mouth and the nose to prevent the transmission of airborne microorganisms.
- Emphasize the need for proper immunizations of all family members.
- For patients with wound care:
  - Teach patient and family signs of wound healing and wound infections.
  - Explain proper technique for changing the dressing and disposing of the soiled ones. Reinforce the need to place contaminated dressings and other disposable items containing body fluids in moisture-proof plastic bags.
  - Have the patient and his or her family repeat instructions and demonstrate skills.
  - If self-injections are required, advise the patient to put used needles in a puncture-resistant container with a screw-top lid. Label so it will not be discarded in the garbage.

SAFE PRACTICE ALERTS!

- Hand hygiene is the most effective method to prevent hospital-acquired infections.
- Drug-resistant microorganisms pose a considerable health risk for both the general population and health care workers. Appropriate use of personal protective equipment (PPE) and hand washing can decrease the risk of transmission.
- Never recap a dirty or used needle because this increases the risk of exposure to blood-borne pathogens.

CHAPTER 23

Hygiene and Patient Care

INDICATIONS FOR HAND HYGIENE[1]

- When hands are visibly dirty or contaminated.
- Before and after having direct contact with patients.
- Before donning sterile gloves.
- When inserting a central intravascular catheter.
- Before inserting indwelling urinary catheters, peripheral vascular catheters, or other invasive devices.
- After contact with a patient's intact skin.
- After contact with body fluids or excretions, mucous membranes, nonintact skin, and wound dressings if hands are not visibly soiled.
- If moving from a contaminated body site to a clean body site during patient care.
- After contact with inanimate objects (including medical equipment) in the immediate vicinity of the patient.
- After removing gloves.
- Before eating and after using a restroom.

---

[1]From CDC guidelines for hand hygiene, 2014, *www.cdc.gov/handhygiene*.

REASONS FOR BATHING[2]

Cleanse the skin: Bathing helps to remove dirt, perspiration, sebum, some bacteria, and dead skin cells. Daily cleaning helps to prevent irritations and rashes that would otherwise transform into infections.

Stimulate blood circulation: Circulation is increased with the use of warm water and gentle stroking of the skin. A person can be relaxed or invigorated through the washing process.

Improve self-image: Bathing promotes a feeling of being refreshed and comfortable. It helps to maintain an acceptable social standard of cleanliness, both appearance and olfactory.

Reduce body odors: Excessive secretion of sweat causes unpleasant body odors. Bathing and use of antiperspirants minimize odors.

Promote range of motion: Movement of the upper and lower extremities during bathing maintains joint function.

TIPS ON GIVING A BED BATH

- Offer a urinal or bedpan, if required, before bed bathing.
- Prepare all items before bath, ensuring they are in easy reach.
- Be sure the water temperature is comfortable for the patient.
- Do *not* rush the bath.
- Allow the patient to participate as much as possible.
- Talk to the patient, to reduce embarrassment and increase comfort.

---

[2]From Yoost BL, Crawford LR: *Fundamentals of nursing: Active learning for collaborative practice*, St. Louis, 2016, Mosby.

- Ensure that the fan or air-conditioning is switched off to prevent the patient from feeling chilled.
- Change the water as needed.
- Begin with face and work down the body.
- Dry the areas immediately.
- Pay special attention to the skin folds, particularly those beneath the breasts, in the groin, and between the buttocks and between the toes.
- Complete a skin assessment during the bath.
- Massage pressure areas, using a firm circular motion.
- Apply nonscented or patient's favorite lotion.
- Perform range of motion during the bath.

A MASSAGE TECHNIQUE
- Assess if massage is contraindicated.
- Start with the patient lying flat or on his or her side.
- Begin with the forehead and work down the body.
- Use a gentle but firm touch.
- Always stroke toward the heart.
- Rub downward on the chest and back.
- Stroke upward on the arms.
- Use a light lotion or oil.

CONTACT LENS CARE
Do
- Wash and rinse hands thoroughly before handling a lens.
- Keep fingernails clean and short.
- Remove lenses from the storage case one at a time and place on the eye.
- Start with the same lens (left or right) every time of insertion.
- Use lens placement technique learned from an eye specialist.

- Use proper lens care products.
- Wear lenses daily and follow the prescribed wearing schedule.
- Remove a lens if it becomes uncomfortable.
- Keep regular appointments with the eye specialist.
- Remove lenses during sunbathing, showering, and swimming.

Do Not
- Use soaps that contain cream or perfume for cleaning lenses.
- Let fingernails touch lenses.
- Mix up lenses.
- Exceed prescribed wearing time.
- Use saliva to wet lenses.
- Use homemade saline solution or tap water to wet or clean lenses.
- Borrow lens solution from another person.

SAFE PRACTICE ALERTS!
- Patients with peripheral neuropathy may not be able to feel the water temperature on their extremities. It is the nurse's responsibility to adjust the bath or shower water to a comfortably warm temperature, 40.5° to 43.3° C (105° to 110° F).
- Always wash the female patient from the urinary meatus back to the anus to prevent introducing organisms into the urinary tract.
- Patients on anticoagulants should use a soft-bristled toothbrush and an electric razor.
- Always have suction equipment at the bedside of comatose patients or patients with decreased gag reflex during oral care.

CHAPTER 24

Activity, Immobility, and Safe Movement

EFFECTS OF IMMOBILITY

- **Musculoskeletal system:** Weakness, decreased muscle tone, decreased bone and muscle mass, potential muscle atrophy and contractures.
- **Nervous system:** Decreased proprioception and balance.
- **Cardiopulmonary system:** Cardiac workload is increased, lung expansion is decreased, pooling of secretions in the lungs, circulatory stasis, risk for deep vein thrombosis, postural or orthostatic hypotension, activity intolerance.
- **Nutrition:** Protein breakdown leading to negative nitrogen balance, anorexia.
- **Elimination:** Urinary stasis, risk for renal calculi, hypomotility of bowel, constipation.
- **Skin:** Necrosis, pressure ulcers.
- **Psychosocial:** Sensory deprivation, sleep disruption, anxiety.

ASSESSMENT QUESTIONS RELATED TO MOBILITY

- Are you experiencing any stiffness, joint discomfort, or pain with movement?
- Have you noticed any difficulty with dizziness or balance?
- Do you become short of breath or easily fatigued when completing your activities of daily living?
- How is your appetite? What is your typical dietary intake in a day?
- What is the frequency of your bowel movements?
- Describe your normal sleep pattern.

EXERCISE

- **Isotonic exercise** involves active movement with constant muscle contraction. Examples include walking, turning in bed, and self-feeding.
- **Isometric exercise** requires tension and relaxation of muscles without joint movement. An example is tension and relaxation of pelvic floor muscles (Kegel exercise).
- **Aerobic exercise** requires oxygen metabolism to produce energy. Patients may engage in rigorous walking or repeated climbing of stairs to achieve the positive effects of aerobic exercise.
- **Anaerobic exercise** builds power and body mass. Without oxygen to produce energy for activity, anaerobic exercise takes place. Heavy weight lifting is an example of anaerobic exercise.

HOME CARE ASSESSMENT[1]

When patients are discharged to home, their activity and exercise need to continue in order to prevent significant skin breakdown and psychosocial isolation.

---

[1]From Yoost BL, Crawford LR: *Fundamentals of nursing: Active learning for collaborative practice*, St. Louis, 2016, Mosby.

- Is the patient able to move independently, or is it necessary for a caregiver to reposition the patient on a scheduled frequency?
- Are preventive skin care measures in place for patients confined to bed?
- Does a pressure-reducing mattress need to be ordered for the patient's home convalescence?
- How often are caregivers or other support people visiting or scheduled to visit and provide diversional activities for the homebound patient?
- Are referrals to community agencies in place to support the homebound patient?

GENERAL PRINCIPLES OF BODY MECHANICS

- Keep the spine in natural alignment while lifting or transferring.
- Elevate work surfaces to approximately elbow height close to the body's center of gravity.
- Never lift more than 35 pounds independently; use additional caregivers and/or mechanical lifts, when appropriate.
- Work with gravity whenever possible.
- Push rather than pull patients or objects.
- Bend from the knees rather than the waist when lifting.
- Avoid twisting while lifting by keeping feet apart with one foot placed in the direction of a transfer.
- Keep patients or objects close to the body to minimize reach.
- Diminish friction and shear by using friction-reducing devices during transfers and having patients lay their arms across their chest during repositioning.
- Use safe patient handling and movement algorithms for decision making in all patient transfers.

JOINT MOVEMENTS

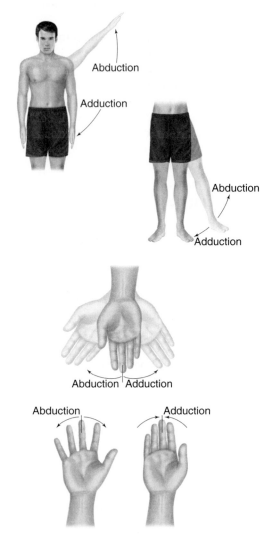

RANGE OF MOTION

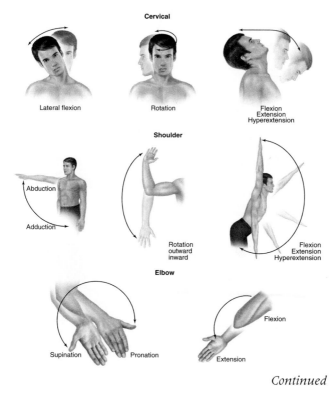

Cervical

Lateral flexion

Rotation

Flexion
Extension
Hyperextension

Shoulder

Abduction

Adduction

Rotation
outward
inward

Flexion
Extension
Hyperextension

Elbow

Supination   Pronation

Flexion

Extension

Continued

RANGE OF MOTION—cont'd

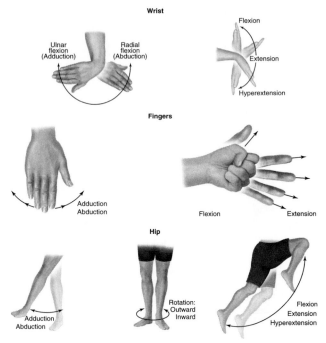

Wrist

Ulnar flexion (Adduction)

Radial flexion (Abduction)

Flexion

Extension

Hyperextension

Fingers

Adduction
Abduction

Flexion

Extension

Hip

Adduction
Abduction

Rotation:
Outward
Inward

Flexion
Extension
Hyperextension

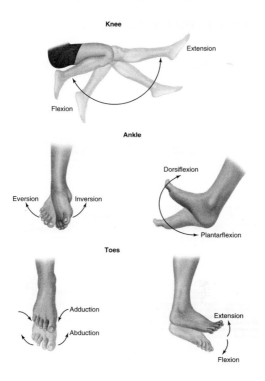

PATIENT POSITIONING

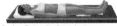

Supine: Patient lies flat on back

Prone: Patient lies face-down

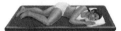

Semi-Fowler: Patient semisitting with head elevated

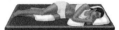

Fowler: Patient in sitting position with pillow supporting thigh and legs

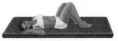

Sims: Patient in semiprone position lying on side

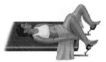

Side-lying: Patient lying on side

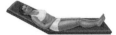

Dorsal recumbent: Patient lying supine with legs bent

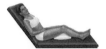

Lithotomy: Patient lying supine

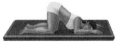

Knee-chest: Patient lying in prone position with buttocks and knees drawn to the chest

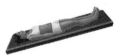

Trendelenburg: Patient lying supine with legs elevated higher than head

SAFE PRACTICE ALERTS!

- Stop range-of-motion exercises if the patient begins to complain of pain or if resistance to movement is experienced. Never hyperextend or flex a patient's joints beyond their position of comfort.
- Assess patients for dizziness and their ability to stand unassisted before allowing ambulation.
- Monitor patient vital signs and stability with position changes when narcotic analgesics are prescribed for pain relief. Adverse side effects of narcotics include confusion, sedation, and dizziness.
- Position patients so that pressure is minimized on all bony prominences.

CHAPTER 25

Skin Integrity and Wound Care

COMMON INTEGUMENTARY ABNORMALITIES

Type	Characteristics	Assess for
Edema	Fluid accumulation	Trauma, murmur, third heart sound
Diaphoresis	Sweating	Pain, fever, anxiety, insulin reaction

Continued

Type	Characteristics	Assess for
Bromhidrosis	Foul perspiration	Infection, poor hygiene
Hirsutism	Hair growth	Adrenal function
Petechiae	Red or purple spots	Hepatic function, drug reactions
Alopecia	Hair loss	Hypopituitarism, medications, fever, starvation

COMMON SKIN COLOR ABNORMALITIES

Type	Characteristics
Albinism	Decreased pigmentation
Vitiligo	White patches on exposed areas
Mongolian spots	Black and blue spots on back and buttocks
Jaundice	Yellow pigmentation of skin or sclera
Ecchymosis	Black and blue marks; assess for trauma, bleeding time, or hepatic function
Cyanosis	Bluish color of lips, earlobes, or nails; assess lung and heart status

NAIL BED ASSESSMENT

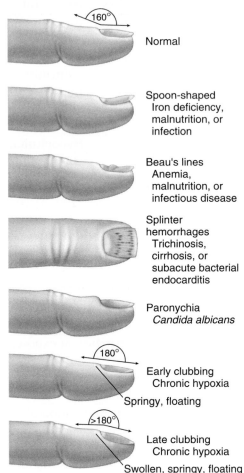

Normal

Spoon-shaped
  Iron deficiency,
  malnutrition, or
  infection

Beau's lines
  Anemia,
  malnutrition, or
  infectious disease

Splinter
hemorrhages
  Trichinosis,
  cirrhosis, or
  subacute bacterial
  endocarditis

Paronychia
  Candida albicans

Early clubbing
  Chronic hypoxia
Springy, floating

Late clubbing
  Chronic hypoxia
Swollen, springy, floating

Abnormalities of the nail bed. (From Harkreader H: *Fundamentals of nursing: Caring and clinical judgment,* ed. 3, St. Louis, 2007, Mosby.)

COMMON FOOT PROBLEMS

Dry skin can cause itching and burning feet. Use mild soap in small amounts and a cream or lotion on your legs and feet every day.

Corns and calluses are caused by pressure when the bony parts of the feet rub against shoes. Wearing shoes that fit better or using nonmedicated pads may help. Use a pumice stone to help reduce the size. Do not try to shave off the corn or callus.

Warts are skin growths caused by viruses. They may be painful and can spread if not treated.

Bunions are swollen and tender joints that can develop at the base of the big toe. Wearing shoes cut wide at the toes may help. Padding the bunion may bring relief.

Ingrown toenails are caused by a piece of the nail piercing the skin. This can happen if the toenails are not cut straight across so the corner of the nail can be seen above the skin.

Neuromas are the result of a buildup of tissue around an inflamed nerve in the foot. Shoes that are too narrow or have high heels can make the problem worse.

Hammertoe is caused by a shortening of the tendons that control toe movements. More space in the shoe or stocking can help.

Spurs are bony bumps that grow on bones of the feet. Standing for long periods of time, wearing badly fitting shoes, or being overweight can make spurs worse. Treatments for spurs include foot supports, heel pads, and heel cups.

Swollen feet may happen after standing for a long time. If the feet and ankles stay swollen, it may be a sign of a more serious health problem.

Fungal infections, such as athlete's foot, happen because the feet are in shoes most of the time. Shoes are warm, dark, and moist. A fungus can cause dry skin, redness, blisters, itching, and peeling. It can be hard to cure. To prevent infections:

- Keep feet clean and dry. Be sure to dry the area between the toes.
- Change shoes and socks or stockings often to help keep feet dry.
- Do not wear tight shoes.
- Try dusting the feet every day with talc-free foot powder.

ORTHOPEDIC DEVICES

Orthopedic devices include a wide range of supports and other devices that are generally used to help support a joint and stabilize areas of the body. Orthotic devices usually limit or prevent movement or hold a body part in a certain position so that further injury or deformation is prevented and healthy and normal development can occur. Orthotic devices are often used to do the following:

- Control, guide, limit, and/or immobilize an extremity, joint, or body segment for a particular reason.
- Restrict movement in a given direction.
- Assist movement generally.
- Reduce weight-bearing forces for a particular purpose.
- Aid rehabilitation from fractures after the removal of a cast.
- Otherwise correct the shape and/or function of the body, to provide easier movement capability or reduce pain.

CMS ASSESSMENT
Circulation (Four Components)

- Color of skin by comparing with unaffected extremity.
- Temperature by feeling both extremities simultaneously.

- Capillary refill by compressing the thumb for a few seconds until it blanches (turns white). Note the return of color. Blood return should be immediate or less than 3 seconds.
- Peripheral pulse noting presence and strength. Compare the pulse with the opposite extremity.

Motor
- Ask patient to move all of the involved fingers or toes.
- Assess for the presence of pain with the movement.

Sensation
- Ask patient about the presence or absence of sensation (e.g., numbness, tingling, or inability to feel pain).
- Pinch each finger or toe and ask the patient to identify which one you are pinching (ask the patient to close his or her eyes for this).
- Note degree of swelling if edema is present.

HEALTH ASSESSMENT QUESTIONS
- Are you able to bathe yourself?
- How often do you bathe or shower?
- Has there been a change in your ability to care for yourself?
- Can you reach your feet and legs when you bathe or shower?
- Are you ever incontinent of urine or stool?
- Do you become short of breath during your bath?
- Can you raise your arms up to brush your teeth?
- Are you able to shampoo and comb your hair?

THE HEALING PROCESS
- **Primary intention:** Edges of wound brought together to heal. *Example:* Surgical incision.
- **Secondary intention:** New tissue fills in from bottom and sides of wound. *Example:* Diabetic foot ulcer.

- **Tertiary intention:** Delay between injury and closure of wound.

PHASES OF WOUND HEALING
- **Inflammatory phase:** Initial response to wound in skin.
- **Proliferative phase:** Repair of wound with granulation tissue.
- **Maturation phase:** Scar tissue forms and strengthens.

FACTORS AFFECTING WOUND HEALING
Age: The very young and very old will generally have longer healing times.

Infection: If an infection is present, as evidenced by purulent drainage or exudate, healing will be delayed.

Hydration: A moist environment allows wounds to heal faster and less painfully than a dry environment.

Nutrition: Poor diet, especially a diet lacking in protein, will delay healing.

Maceration: Urinary and fecal incontinence can alter the skin's integrity and delay healing.

Necrosis: Dead, devitalized (necrotic) tissue can delay healing.

Pressure: When pressure at the wound site is excessive or sustained, the blood supply to the capillary network may be disrupted. This impedes blood flow to the surrounding tissue and delays healing.

Trauma: Wounds heal slowly—and may not heal at all—in an environment in which they are repeatedly traumatized or deprived of local blood supply by edema.

Chronic diseases: Coronary artery disease, peripheral vascular disease, cancer, and diabetes mellitus are a few of the chronic diseases that can compromise wound healing.

Immunosuppression and radiation therapy: Suppression of the immune system by disease, medication, or age can delay wound healing.

COMPLICATIONS OF WOUND HEALING

Dehiscence: A partial or complete separation of the tissue layers during the healing process.

Evisceration: A total separation of the tissue layers allowing the protrusion of visceral organs through the incision.

Fistulas: Abnormal connections between two internal organs or between an internal organ and the outside of the body through the skin.

Pressure ulcer: A localized injury to the skin and/or underlying tissue usually over a bony prominence, as a result of pressure, or pressure in combination with shear.

CLASSIFICATION OF PRESSURE ULCERS

Stage I: Intact, nonblistered skin with nonblanchable erythema, or persistent redness in an area that has been exposed to pressure.

Stage II: Partial-thickness wound that involves the epidermis and/or dermis but does not extend below the level of the dermis.

Stage III: Full-thickness wounds that extend into the subcutaneous tissue but do not extend through the fascia to muscle, bone, or connective tissue.

Stage IV: Deeper than a stage III pressure ulcer and there is exposure of muscle, bone, or connective tissues, such as tendons or cartilage.

Unstageable: Wound is a full-thickness wound where the wound bed contains enough necrotic tissue or eschar that it is not possible to assess the depth of the wound or the involvement of underlying structures.

SITES OF PRESSURE ULCERS

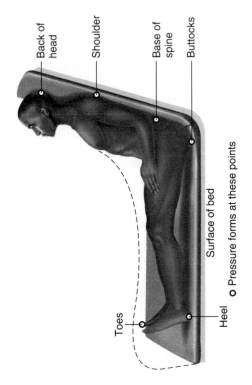

Back of head

Shoulder

Base of spine

Buttocks

Surface of bed

o Pressure forms at these points

Toes

Heel

BRADEN SCALE

BRADEN SCALE FOR PREDICTING PRESSURE SORE RISK

Patient's Name _____ Evaluator's Name _____ Date of Assessment _____

SENSORY PERCEPTION Ability to respond meaningfully to pressure-related discomfort	**1. Completely Limited** Unresponsive (does not moan, flinch, or grasp) to painful stimuli, due to diminished level of consciousness or sedation. OR Limited ability to feel pain over most of body.	**2. Very Limited** Responds only to painful stimuli. Cannot communicate discomfort except by moaning or restlessness. OR Has a sensory impairment which limits the ability to feel pain or discomfort over ½ of body.	**3. Slightly Limited** Responds to verbal commands, but cannot always communicate discomfort or the need to be turned. OR Has some sensory impairment which limits the ability to feel pain or discomfort in 1 or 2 extremities.	**4. No Impairment** Responds to verbal commands. Has no sensory deficit which limits ability to feel or voice pain and discomfort.
MOISTURE Degree to which skin is exposed to moisture	**1. Constantly Moist** Skin is kept moist almost constantly by perspiration, urine, etc. Dampness is detected every time patient is moved or turned.	**2. Very Moist** Skin is often, but not always moist. Linen must be changed at least once a shift.	**3. Occasionally Moist** Skin is occasionally moist, requiring an extra linen change approximately once a day.	**4. Rarely Moist** Skin is usually dry, linen only requires changing at routine intervals.
ACTIVITY Degree of physical activity	**1. Bedfast** Confined to bed.	**2. Chairfast** Ability to walk severely limited or non-existent. Cannot bear own weight and/or must be assisted into chair or wheelchair.	**3. Walks Occasionally** Walks occasionally during day, but for very short distances, with or without assistance. Spends majority of each shift in bed or chair.	**4. Walks Frequently** Walks outside room at least twice a day and inside room at least once every 2 hours during waking hours.
MOBILITY Ability to change and control body position	**1. Completely Immobile** Does not make even slight changes in body or extremity position without assistance.	**2. Very Limited** Makes occasional slight changes in body or extremity position but unable to make frequent or significant changes independently.	**3. Slightly Limited** Makes frequent though slight changes in body or extremity position independently.	**4. No Limitation** Makes major and frequent changes in position without assistance.
NUTRITION Usual food intake pattern	**1. Very Poor** Never eats a complete meal. Rarely eats more than ⅓ of any food offered. Eats 2 servings or less of protein (meat or dairy products) per day. Takes fluids poorly. Does not take a liquid dietary supplement. OR Is NPO and/or maintained on clear liquids or IV's for more than 5 days.	**2. Probably Inadequate** Rarely eats a complete meal and generally eats only about ½ of any food offered. Protein intake includes only 3 servings of meat or dairy products per day. Occasionally will take a dietary supplement. OR Receives less than optimum amount of liquid diet or tube feeding.	**3. Adequate** Eats over half of most meals. Eats a total of 4 servings of protein (meat, dairy products) per day. Occasionally will refuse a meal, but will usually take a supplement when offered. OR Is on a tube feeding or TPN regimen which probably meets most of nutritional needs.	**4. Excellent** Eats most of every meal. Never refuses a meal. Usually eats a total of 4 or more servings of meat and dairy products. Occasionally eats between meals. Does not require supplementation.
FRICTION & SHEAR	**1. Problem** Requires moderate to maximum assistance in moving. Complete lifting without sliding against sheets is impossible. Frequently slides down in bed or chair requiring frequent repositioning with maximum assistance. Spasticity, contractures, or agitation leads to almost constant friction.	**2. Potential Problem** Moves freely or requires minimum assistance. During a move, skin probably slides to some extent against sheets, chair restraints or other devices. Maintains relatively good position in chair or bed most of the time but occasionally slides down.	**3. No Apparent Problem** Moves in bed and in chair independently and has sufficient muscle strength to lift up completely during move. Maintains good position in bed or chair.	

Total Score _____

(Adapted from Barbara Braden, PhD, RN, Creighton University School of Nursing, Omaha, Nebraska.)

SAFE PRACTICE ALERTS!

- Remove products with a strong adhesive backing, such as found in tapes and adhesive dressings, carefully in the elderly to prevent stripping off the epidermis.
- Wound irrigation can result in splashing of the fluid and debris, therefore the use of personal protective equipment such as gowns, masks, and goggles is required.
- Warm compresses and water for soaks should not be heated in the microwave unless the product and microwave are specifically designed for this type of heating. The uneven heating and inability to measure the resultant temperature can result in serious burns to the patient.

CHAPTER 26

Nutrition

TYPES OF DIETS

Type	Description	Patient Issue
Regular	Has all essentials; no restrictions	No special diet needed
Clear liquid	Broth, tea, clear soda, strained juices, gelatin	Recovery from surgery or very ill
Full liquid	Clear liquids plus milk products, eggs	Transition from clear to regular diet
Soft	Soft consistency and mild spice	Difficulty swallowing
Mechanical soft	Regular diet but chopped or ground	Difficulty chewing

Continued

199

TYPES OF DIETS—cont'd

Type	Description	Patient Issue
Bland	No spicy food	Ulcers or colitis
Low residue	No bulky food, apples, or nuts	Rectal disease
High calorie	High protein, vitamin, and fat	Malnourished
Low calorie	Decreased fat, no whole milk, cream, eggs, complex carbohydrates	Obese
Diabetic	Balance of protein, carbohydrates, fat	Insulin-food imbalance
High protein	Meat, fish, milk, cheese, poultry, eggs	Tissue repair, underweight
Low fat	Little butter, cream, whole milk, or eggs	Gallbladder, liver, or heart disease
Low cholesterol	Little meat or cheese	Need to decrease fat intake
Low sodium	No salt added during cooking	Heart or renal disease
Salt free	No salt	Heart or renal disease
Tube feeding	Formulas or liquid food	Oral surgery, oral or esophageal cancers, inability to eat or swallow

THERAPEUTIC DIETS

Clear liquid: Limited nutrients; only used for a
short period of time. Clear juices that do not
contain pulp. Examples: apple or cranberry juice,
gelatin, popsicles, and clear broths. Prescribed
for patients with gastrointestinal (GI) problems,
before (preoperatively) and after surgery.
(postoperatively), and before some diagnostic tests.

Full liquid: Foods that are or may become liquid
at room or body temperature. Examples: juices
(including those with pulp), milk and milk
products, yogurt, strained cream soups, and
liquid dietary supplements. Used to advance a
patient with GI disturbances, after having dental
work performed, and for those patients who
cannot tolerate solid food.

Pureed: Food is placed into a blender and made
into a pulp-like mixture. This type of diet is used
for persons who cannot safely chew or swallow
solid food. The addition of raw eggs, nuts, and
seeds should be avoided.

Mechanical soft: Food consistencies that have
been modified such as ground meat or soft
cooked foods. They are also used for persons who
have difficulty chewing effectively.

Thickened liquids: Used for patients who
have difficulty swallowing and are at risk for
aspiration. Liquids are thickened by adding a
commercially prepared thickening agent. Avoid
nuts, seeds, and other hard or raw foods to
decrease the risk of aspiration.

Regular/general: There are no dietary restrictions.
The diet is intended to supply patients with a
balanced diet of essential nutrients.

Diabetes (ADA): Prescribed to control the
amount of calories by controlling the
carbohydrate intake. Avoid high glycemic

index foods that raise the body's blood glucose concentration rapidly. Complex carbohydrates from vegetables and fruits are preferred to simple carbohydrates, sugars, and starchy foods, such as bread or pie.

Cardiac: Used to control the dietary intake of certain foods that contribute to conditions that affect the cardiovascular system. They typically consist of low cholesterol and low sodium dietary items. Cardiac diets minimize the intake of animal products, which contain cholesterol, and soups and processed foods such as pickles and lunch meats, which are high in sodium.

Renal: Restrict potassium, sodium, protein, and phosphorus intake. Fresh fruits (except bananas) and vegetables are excellent dietary choices for individuals on a renal diet. Meats, processed foods, peanut butter, cheese, nuts, caramels, ice cream, and colas are typically allowed in limited quantities or contraindicated.

NUTRIENTS

Type	Function	Food Sources
Carbohydrate	Energy, body temperature	*Simple:* Sugars, fruits, nuts *Complex:* Grains, potatoes, milk
Protein	Tissue growth, tissue repair	Complete: Meat, fish, eggs, milk, poultry, beans, peas, nuts

Type	Function	Food Sources
Fat	Energy and repair, carries vitamins A and D	Incomplete: Animal fat, meat, nuts, milk, fish, poultry, vegetables, breads
Water	Carries nutrients, regulates body processes, lubricates joints, maintain acid-base balance	Liquids, most fruits and vegetables

VITAMINS

Type	Function	Food Sources
A (retinol)	Helps eyes, skin, hair, bones, and teeth; fights infection	Yellow fruits and vegetables, liver, kidneys, fish
B_1 (thiamine)	Maintains nerves, aids carbohydrate function	Bread, cereal, beans, peas, pork, liver, eggs, milk
B_2 (riboflavin)	Maintains skin, mouth, nerve functions, metabolism of protein	Dairy, cheese, eggs, cereal, dark green vegetables, whole grains
B_3 (niacin)	Oxidation of proteins and carbohydrates, formation of fatty acids	Meat, fish, poultry, eggs, nuts, bread, cereal, dried beans, whole grains
B_5 (pantothenic acid)	Metabolism of carbohydrates, fats, and proteins	Whole grain cereals, potatoes, legumes, broccoli
B_6 (pyridoxine)	Synthesis of amino acids	Spinach, squash, bell peppers

B_9 (folic acid)	Synthesis of DNA, red blood cell formation, rapidly growing cells	Green vegetables, oranges, strawberries, dried beans, peas/nuts, enriched breads
B_{12} (cyanocobalamin)	Aids muscles, nerves, heart, metabolism	Organ meats, milk
Biotin	Forms DNA and RNA	Liver, legumes, tomatoes, egg yolk
C (ascorbic acid)	Maintains integrity of cells, repairs tissue, synthesizes collagen	Citrus fruits, tomatoes, green vegetables, potatoes
D	Enables body to use calcium and phosphorus	Dairy, margarine, fish, liver, eggs
F	Antioxidant, protects immune system	Peanuts, vegetable oils
K	Aids in blood clotting	Dark green leafy vegetables

MINERALS

Type	Function	Food Sources
Calcium	Renews bones and teeth, regulates heart and nerves	Milk, green vegetables, cheese, salmon, legumes
Phosphorus	Renews bones and teeth, maintains nerve function	Cheese, oats, meat, milk, fish, poultry, nuts
Iron	Renews hemoglobin	Meat, eggs, liver, flour, yellow or green vegetables
Iodine	Regulates thyroid	Table salt, seafood
Magnesium	Component of enzymes	Grains, green vegetables
Sodium	Maintains water balance, nerve function	Salt, cured meats
Potassium	Maintains nerve function	Meat, milk, vegetables
Chloride	Formation of gastric juices	Salt
Zinc	Component of enzymes	Meat, seafood

MALNUTRITION

Marasmus: Caused by decreased caloric intake.
- Takes months to years to develop.
- Individuals appear thin and malnourished.
- Weight loss present.
- Serum albumin and transferrin levels normal.
- Mortality rate low unless from underlying disease.

Kwashiorkor: Lack of protein intake accompanied by fluid retention.

Anorexia: Loss of appetite from suppressed desire to eat.

Anorexia nervosa: Eating disorder resulting in significant weight loss and health risk.

Bulimia nervosa: Eating disorder consisting of food binging (intake) and purging (vomiting).

SAFE PRACTICE ALERTS!
- Do not attempt to feed food or liquids to a patient in a supine position. The head of the bed must be elevated 30 to 45 degrees with the patient in an upright position to minimize the risk for aspiration. Have a suction machine at the bedside at all times.

CHAPTER 27

Cognitive and Sensory Alterations

SENSORY DEFICITS

Tactile: Damage to sensory nerve fibers leads to peripheral neuropathy. Patients may not be able to feel sharp objects or discern extreme hot and cold temperatures, leaving them vulnerable to injury.

Smell: The ability to smell can decrease with age. Infections, smoking, and cocaine use can also damage ability to smell.

Taste: The ability to taste can decrease with age. Dentures; injury to the tongue, cheeks, or roof of the mouth; or many medications can damage or change the ability to taste.

Hearing: Otitis media and blockage can cause conductive hearing loss. Persistent exposure to loud noises, adverse reaction to ototoxic drugs, head injuries, or certain infections cause sensorineural hearing loss, or damage to the receptor nerves or nerve pathways.

Vision:
- **Myopia,** or nearsightedness, causes a person to be able to see clearly only a short distance. This is because the image is focused in front of the retina instead of on the retina. Myopia is corrected through the use of a concave lens or through refractive surgery.
- **Presbyopia,** or farsightedness, is a decrease in the ability to focus on near objects. Reading lenses correct presbyopia.
- **Cataracts** are the clouding of the lens of the eye. The clouded lens is removed, and a new lens is placed in the eye.
- **Glaucoma** is an increased intraocular pressure, which puts pressure on the optic nerve, leading to loss of peripheral visual fields and possibly blindness.
- **Macular degeneration** decreases the central visual fields.

Equilibrium: Motion sickness is a common equilibrium problem associated with mixed signals that the brain is receiving. If a person is in a moving object, such as an airplane, boat, or car, and sees only stationary objects, such as the seat in front of the person, the eye is seeing stillness while the inner ear is detecting movement. The symptoms are dizziness, nausea, and vomiting.

SENSORY AIDS AND INTERVENTIONS
- Orient by using clock, calendar, use of familiar objects.
- Keep environment free of clutter, bright lights, loud noises.
- Call light within reach.
- Pressure-sensitive alarms.
- Face patient.
- Monitor water temperature to maintain safety.

- Encourage well-balanced diet with various textures and aromas.
- Maintain glasses and/or hearing aids in clean, working order.
- Keep walkways clear, assist as needed with ambulation.
- Use nonskid footwear.

ASSESSING PATIENT'S SENSORY AIDS
Eyeglasses
- Purpose for wearing glasses (e.g., reading distance, or both).
- Methods used to clean glasses.
- Presence of symptoms (e.g., blurred vision, photophobia, headaches, irritation).

Contact Lenses
- Type of lenses worn.
- Frequency and duration of time lenses are worn (including sleep time).
- Presence of symptoms (e.g., burning, excess tearing, redness, irritation, swelling, sensitivity to light).
- Techniques used by the patient to clean, store, insert, and remove lenses.
- Use of eyedrops or ointments.
- Use of emergency identification bracelet or card that warns others to remove patient's lenses in case of emergency.

Artificial Eye
- Method used to insert and remove eye.
- Method for cleaning eye.
- Presence of symptoms (e.g., drainage, inflammation, pain involving the orbit).

Hearing Aid
- Type of aid worn.
- Methods used to clean aid.

COMPARISON OF DELIRIUM AND DEMENTIA

Feature	Delirium	Dementia
Onset	Rapid, often at night	Usually insidious
Duration	Hours to weeks	Months to years
Course	Fluctuates over 24 hr	Relatively stable
		Worse at night
		Lucid intervals
Awareness	Always impaired	Usually normal
Alertness	Fluctuates	Usually normal
Orientation	Impaired; often will mistake people or places	May be intact May confabulate
Memory	Recent and immediate memory impaired	Recent and remote memory impaired
Thinking	Slow, accelerated, or dreamlike	Poor in abstraction Impoverished
Perception	Often misperceives	Becomes absent
Sleep cycle	Disrupted at night Drowsiness during day	Fragmented sleep
Physical	Often sick	Often well at first

DEPRESSION
Minor depression: At least two of the following symptoms.

Major depression: At least five of the following symptoms.

Dysthymia (chronic depression): Symptoms exist over at least 2 years.

Assessment areas:

- Dysphoria—depressed mood (irritability in some people).
- Loss of pleasure or interest.
- Change in appetite and weight.
- Insomnia or hypersomnia.
- Psychomotor agitation or retardation.
- Fatigue or loss of energy.
- Feelings of worthlessness and/or excessive guilt.
- Decreased ability to concentrate, think, or make decisions.
- Recurrent thoughts of death, suicidal ideation.

SAFE PRACTICE ALERTS!

- The nurse ensures the safety of hospitalized patients with visual changes by telling the patient about the room environment and describing the location of needed objects. As with all patients, it is imperative that the patient has a call light within reach.
- Communication is key to all nursing interactions. Modifications are made for patients with communication deficits to enable meaningful communication.

CHAPTER 28

Stress and Coping

FIGHT-OR-FLIGHT RESPONSE

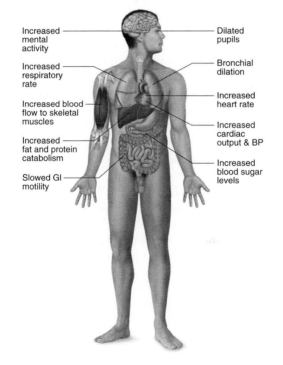

Increased mental activity

Increased respiratory rate

Increased blood flow to skeletal muscles

Increased fat and protein catabolism

Slowed GI motility

Dilated pupils

Bronchial dilation

Increased heart rate

Increased cardiac output & BP

Increased blood sugar levels

DEFENSE MECHANISMS[1]

A defense mechanism is a technique of coping that helps to reduce anxiety generated by threats from unacceptable or negative impulses.

Compensation: Focusing on strengths rather than perceived weaknesses.

Denial: Ignoring aspects of reality that induce anxiety or contribute to a loss of self-esteem.

Displacement: Redirecting negative emotions perceived as unacceptable or threatening to a safer focus.

Intellectualization: Overthinking a challenging situation or impulse to avoid dealing with the emotions it elicits.

Projection: Attributing one's own motives, values, desires, situational responses, and personality traits to another person.

Rationalization: Explaining personal actions in such a way as to enhance one's own self-image.

Regression: Reverting to behavior associated with an earlier stage of development when challenged by thoughts and stressors.

Repression: Blocking unacceptable thoughts and feelings from consciousness.

STRESS MANAGEMENT TECHNIQUES

Stress management starts with identifying the sources of stress. Strategies may be helpful for you as a professional or for your patients.

• Keep a stress journal to help identify the regular stressors.
  • Note the causes of the stress and your reactions to the stress.

---

[1]From Yoost BL, Crawford LR: *Fundamentals of nursing: Active learning for collaborative practice,* St. Louis, 2016, Mosby.

- Note what makes the stress worse and what helps to relieve it.
- Reduce caffeine and sugar intake: The temporary "highs" caffeine and sugar provide often end with a crash in mood and energy.
- Nutrition: When people eat a balanced diet they feel better and manage stress better.
- Sleep: When people sleep better they feel better and can handle stress better.
- Relaxation: Use guided imagery, exercise, meditation, mindfulness, yoga, biofeedback.
- Avoid alcohol, cigarettes, and drugs: Self-medicating with alcohol or drugs may provide an easy escape from stress, but the relief is only temporary.

SAFE PRACTICE ALERT!
- Verbalization of suicidal ideation or a plan must be taken seriously. In the case of a hospitalized patient, one-on-one observation should be implemented to ensure patient safety and referral to psychiatric services should be implemented. Do not leave the patient alone.

CHAPTER 29

Sleep

PATIENT'S SLEEP HISTORY
- Have the patient describe his or her specific problem.
- Have the patient describe his or her symptoms and alleviating factors.
- Assess the patient's normal sleep pattern.
- Assess the patient's normal bedtime rituals.
- Assess for current or recent physical illnesses.
- Assess for current or recent emotional stress.
- Assess for possible sleep disorders.
- Assess the patient's current medications and their possible effects on sleep.

SLEEP DISORDERS
- **Insomnia** is trouble initiating or maintaining sleep.
- **Obstructive sleep apnea** is the absence of breathing (apnea) or diminished breathing during sleep between snoring intervals.
- **Hypersomnia** is excessive daytime sleepiness.
- **Restless legs syndrome** is a sleep disorder characterized by disagreeable leg movements resulting from intense, abnormal, lower

extremity sensations of crawling or tingling feelings.

- **Narcolepsy** is the chronic neurologic disorder causing an uncontrollable desire to sleep.
- **Sleep deprivation** is the prolonged, inadequate quality and quantity of sleep.
- **Nocturnal enuresis** is bedwetting at night.
- **Somnambulism** is sleepwalking.
- **Sleep terrors** is when the patient awakens from sleep in a terrified state.
- **Bruxism** is the clenching of the teeth tightly or grinding them from side to side.

FACTORS CAUSING SLEEP ALTERATIONS

- Anxiety and stress are the main causes of short-term sleep problems
- Beverages with caffeine
- Lifestyle factors such as work schedule
- Diet and exercise
- Smoking
- Alcohol use
- Stimulants and other medications
- Environmental factors
- Illness and hospitalization

MEDICATIONS THAT AFFECT SLEEP

Hypnotics

- Interfere with reaching deep sleep stages
- Only temporary increase in quantity of sleep
- May cause "hangover" during day
- Excess drowsiness, confusion, decreased energy
- May worsen sleep apnea in older adults

Diuretics

- Cause nocturia

Antidepressants and Stimulants
- Suppress rapid eye movement (REM) sleep

Alcohol
- Speeds onset of sleep
- Disrupts REM sleep
- May cause awakening from sleep and causes difficulty returning to sleep

Caffeine
- Prevents the person from falling asleep
- May cause awakening from sleep

Nonbenzodiazepines
- Anxiety and irritability
- Sleepwalking, sleep eating, or sleep driving

Digoxin
- Causes nightmares

Beta Blockers
- Cause nightmares
- Cause insomnia
- Cause awakening from sleep

Valium
- Decreases stages 2 and 4 and REM sleep
- Decreases awakenings

Narcotics (Morphine/Meperidine [Demerol])
- Suppress REM sleep
- If discontinued quickly, can increase risk of cardiac dysrhythmias because of "rebound REM" periods
- Cause increased awakenings and drowsiness

SAFE PRACTICE ALERTS!

- Obstructive sleep apnea can cause fragmented sleep and low blood oxygen levels, leading to hypoxia, acidosis, and hypercapnia (increased carbon dioxide) to the body, including the heart.
- When administering medications that affect sleep, be sure beds are in low position, night lights are on, and call lights are within reach to help prevent patient falls. No alcohol products should be ingested with sleeping medications.

Nursing Care

For more in-depth information on nursing basics, consult the following:

Yoost BL, Crawford LR: *Fundamentals of nursing: Active learning for collaborative practice*, St. Louis, 2016, Mosby.

CHAPTER 30

Diagnostic Testing

COMMON DIAGNOSTIC TESTS

Angiography: Records cardiac pressures, function, and output (patient may need special postprocedure vital signs taken).

Antinuclear antibody (ANA): A group of antibodies used to diagnose lupus (SLE).

Arterial blood gases: Measurements of arterial blood pH, PO_2, $PaCO_2$, and bicarbonate. Blood sample needs to be kept on ice.

Arteriography: Radiographic examination with injections of dye used to locate occlusions. Patient may need special postprocedure vital signs taken.

Arthrography: Radiographic examination of the bones.

Arthroscopy: Procedure that allows examination of the joint.

Barium study: Radiographic examination to locate polyps, tumors, or other colon problems. (Barium needs to be removed after procedure).

Barium swallow: Detects esophageal narrowing, varices, strictures, or tumors. (Barium needs to be removed after procedure).

Biopsy: Removal of specific tissue. Assess patient for pain after procedure.

Blood tests: See following section on Laboratory Values for normal values.

Bone densitometry: Test to determine bone mineral content and density; used to diagnose osteoporosis.

Bone marrow biopsy: Examination of a piece of tissue from bone marrow. Assess patient for pain after procedure.

Bone scan: Used to locate tumors or other bone disorders. Patient must be able to lie flat.

Brain scan: Used to locate tumors, strokes, or seizure disorders. Patient must be able to lie flat.

Bronchoscopy: Inspection of the larynx, trachea, and bronchi with flexible scope. Patient may need sedation.

Cardiac catheterization: Uses dye to visualize the heart's arteries. Patient may need special postprocedure vital signs taken.

Chest radiographs: Used to look for pneumonia, cancer, and other diseases of the lung.

Cholangiography: Radiographic examination of the biliary ducts.

Cholecystography: Radiographic examination of the gallbladder.

Colonoscopy: Uses flexible scope to view colon. Patient may need to be sedated.

Colposcopy: Examination of the cervix and vagina.

Computed tomography (CT) scan: Three-dimensional radiography. Patient must lie flat.

Culdoscopy: Flexible tube used to view pelvic organs.

Culture and sensitivity: Determines source and type of bacteria.

Cystoscopy: Direct visualization of bladder with cystoscope.

Dilation and curettage: Dilation of the cervix followed by endometrial cleansing.

Doppler: Ultrasonography used to show venous or arterial patency.

Echocardiography: Ultrasonography that records structure and functions of the heart.

Electrocardiography: Records electrical impulses generated by the heart.

Electroencephalography (EEG): Records electrical activity of the brain.

Electromyography (EMG): Records electrical activity of the muscles.

Endoscopy: Inspection of upper gastrointestinal (GI) tract with flexible scope. Patient may need to be sedated.

Endoscopic retrograde cholangiopancreatography (ERCP): Radiographic examination of the gallbladder and pancreas.

Exercise stress test: Recording of the heart rate, activity, and blood pressure while the body is at work.

Fluoroscopy: Radiographic examination with picture displayed on television monitor.

GI series: Radiographic examination using barium to locate ulcers. Barium must be removed after procedure.

Glucose tolerance test (GTT): Determines ability to tolerate an oral glucose load; used to establish diabetes.

Hemoccult: Detects blood in stool, emesis, and elsewhere.

Holter monitor: Checks and records irregular heart rates and rhythms (generally over a 24-hour period).

Intravenous pyelography (IVP): Radiographic examination of the kidneys after dye injection.

KUB: Radiographic examination of the kidneys, ureter, and bladder.

Laparoscopy: Abdominal examination with a flexible scope.

Lumbar puncture: Sampling of spinal fluid, often called a spinal tap (can be done at bedside).

Magnetic resonance imaging (MRI): Three-dimensional radiograph similar to CT scan.

Mammography: Radiographic examination of the breast.

Myelography: Injection of dye into subarachnoid space to view brain and spinal cord.

Oximetry: Method to monitor arterial blood saturation.

Papanicolaou (Pap) smear: Detects cervical cancer.

Proctoscopy: Inspection of lower colon with flexible scope. Patient may need to be sedated.

Pulmonary function test (PFT): Measures lung capacity and volume to detect problems.

Pyelography: Radiographic examination of kidneys.

Sigmoidoscopy: Inspection of lower colon with flexible scope. Patient may need to be sedated.

Small bowel follow-through (SBFT): Done in addition to a GI series.

Spinal tap: See Lumbar puncture.

Thallium: Radionuclear dye used to assess heart functions.

Titer: A blood test to determine the presence of antibodies.

Tuberculin skin test: Test for tuberculosis using tuberculin purified protein derivative (PPD).

Ultrasonography: Reflection of sound waves.

Urine tests: See following section on Laboratory Values for normal values.

Venography: Radiographic examination used to locate a thrombus in a vein.

LABORATORY VALUES

Complete Blood Cell Count	
Value	**Reference Range***
Red blood cells (RBCs)	Males: 4.7-6.1×10 mL
	Females: 4.2-5.4×10 mL
White blood cells (WBCs)	5000-10,000 mm^3
Neutrophils	Adult: 50%-70%
	Child: 30%-60%
Lymphocytes	Adult: 20%-40%
	Child: 25%-50%
Monocytes	3%-8%
Eosinophils	1%-4%
Basophils	0%-1%
Hemoglobin (Hgb)	Males: 14-18 g/dL
	Females: 12-16 g/dL
Hematocrit (Hct)	Males: 42%-52%
	Females: 37%-48%

Coagulation Value	**Reference Range***
Platelet	150,000-400,000 mL
Prothrombin time (PT)	11-12.5 sec

Continued

LABORATORY VALUES—cont'd

Coagulation Value	Reference Range*
Partial thromboplastin time (PTT)	30-45 sec
Thrombin time (TT)	Control ±5 sec
Fibrinogen split products (FSP)	Negative reaction at >1: 4 dilution
Iron or ferritin (Fe) (deficiency)	0-20 ng/mL
Reticulocyte count	0.5-1.5% of RBC

*Ranges may vary by organization.

Blood Chemistry	
Value	Range*
Sodium (Na^+)	135-145 mEq/L
Potassium (K^+)	3.5-5.5 mEq/L
Chloride (Cl^-)	95-112 mEq/L
Anion gap	4-14 mEq/L
Carbon dioxide (CO_2)	24-32 mEq/L
Blood urea nitrogen (BUN)	10-20 mg/dL
Creatinine (Cr)	0.6-1.3 mg/dL Males
	0.5-1.1 mg/dL (females)
Glucose	60-110 mg/dL
Calcium (Ca^{++})	8.5-10.5 mg/dL
Magnesium (Mg)	1.3-2.1 mg/dL
Phosphorus	2.5-4.5 mg/dL
Osmolality	275-295 mOsm/kg

*Ranges may vary by organization.

Liver Function Test

Value	Reference Range*
Aspartate aminotransferase (AST)	0-42 U/L
Alanine aminotransferase (ALT)	Females: 7-30 U/L
	Males: 10-55 U/L
Alkaline phosphatase (ALP)	Adult: 20-125 U/L
	Child: 40-400 U/L
Bilirubin: Direct	0-0.2 mg/dL
Bilirubin: Total	0.3-1.0 mg/lb
Amylase	50-150 U/L
Lipase	0-110 U/L

*Ranges may vary by organization.

Urine Electrolytes

Value	Reference Range*
Sodium (Na^+)	40-220 mEq/L
Potassium (K^+)	25-125 mEq/L
Chloride (Cl^-)	110-250 mEq/L

*Ranges may vary by organization.

Lipids

Value	Reference Range*
Cholesterol	<200 mg/dL
Low-density lipoprotein (LDL)	<130 mg/dL
High-density lipoprotein (HDL)	40-60 mg/dL
Triglycerides	Male: 40-160 mg/dL Female: 35-135 mg/dL
Cholesterol:LDL ratio	1:6-1:4.5

*Ranges may vary by organization.

Thyroid

Value	Reference Range*
Thyroxine (T_4)	4-12 µg/dL
Triiodothyronine (T_3) uptake	27-47%
Thyroid-stimulating hormone (TSH)	0.5-6 mU/L

*Ranges may vary by organization.

Cardiac Enzymes*	
Creatine phosphokinase (CK)	Levels rise 4-8 hr after an acute myocardial infarction (MI), peaking at 16-30 hr and returning to baseline within 4 days (25-200 U/L; 32-150 U/L)
CK-MB CK isoenzyme	Increases 6-10 hr after an acute MI, peaks in 24 hr, and remains elevated for up to 72 hr <12 IU/L if total CK is <400 IU/L 400 IU/L
Lactate dehydrogenase (LDH)	Increases 2-5 days after an MI; the elevation can last 10 days (140-280 U/L)

*Averages may vary per facility.

BLOOD COLLECTION TUBES

Yellow: Used for blood cultures

Light blue/citrate: Used for coagulation studies: PT, PTT, and fibrinogen

Red: Used for most blood chemistries and serology tests and blood bank testing

Red/black: Used for most blood chemistries and serology tests

Green: Used for stat blood chemistries

Lavender/purple/navy: Used for hematology studies

Gray: Used for glucose, blood alcohol levels, and lactic acid

ASSESSMENT QUESTIONS RELATED TO DIAGNOSTIC TESTS[1]

- What medications do you take on a daily basis (include prescription, herbal, and over-the-counter medications)?
- Do you have any allergies to food or medications? What happens if you take them?
- What is your understanding of the test? Do you have any questions?
- What medications did you take before the examination? Prescriptions? Over the counter?
- Have you smoked or consumed alcohol in the past 24 hours?
- For females: Is there any chance that you might be pregnant? When was your last menstrual period?
- What preparation did you make for this test (laxatives, NPO, and so forth)?

NURSING CARE FOR DIAGNOSTIC TESTING

Patient identification: Check for the presence of an identification band. Ensure that the band is on the patient and is correct.

Active order: Review medical record to ensure there is an order for the diagnostic test, ensuring the right patient will have the correct test.

Medical history: Review the medical record for a history of medical disorders that may signal a high risk for complications (bleeding disorders, hypertension, etc.).

Allergies: Check for allergies to food or medications. If the patient is undergoing an exam that involves an iodine contrast medium, check

---

[1]From Yoost BL, Crawford LR: *Fundamentals of nursing: Active learning for collaborative practice,* St. Louis, 2016, Mosby.

for a history of adverse reactions or allergies to iodine-containing food (e.g., shellfish, cabbage, kale, and iodized salt).

Informed consent: Check that the consent form has been signed, dated, and witnessed.

Baseline vitals: Obtain and document a complete set of vital signs. This provides a baseline for comparison during the procedure.

Medications: Consult with the health care provider as to whether regularly scheduled medications should be administered or held before the diagnostic test.

Nutrition: When appropriate, ensure that the patient has maintained NPO status.

Preparations: Determine whether the ordered preparations (e.g., laxatives or cathartics, fluid or antibiotics) were taken by the patient. Document the results.

IV access: If the procedure requires IV access for the administration of medications and/or contrast media, be sure the IV is patent and well secured. Also if preprocedure sedative or analgesic has been ordered, ensure that the medication is given at the appropriate time.

HOME CARE CONSIDERATIONS FOR DIAGNOSTIC TESTING[2]

It is not uncommon for the patient to be asked to collect a specimen at home and transport it to the health care center.

- Does the patient understand the collection instructions? They would include timing of the collection, cleansing procedures, contamination precautions, and so on.

---

[2]From Yoost BL, Crawford LR: *Fundamentals of nursing: Active learning for collaborative practice,* St. Louis, 2016, Mosby.

- Does the patient have the appropriate equipment and containers to collect the specimen?
- How is the specimen to be transported?
- Does it need to be kept warm or cold?
- When does it need to be transported? Immediately or within a few hours?

HOME CARE CONSIDERATIONS FOR GLUCOSE TESTING[3]

Patients with diabetes mellitus are asked to monitor their blood glucose levels on a daily basis at home.

- Does the patient understand the procedure and frequency of testing? A return demonstration is helpful in assessing the patient's level of understanding.
- Are there financial concerns regarding the testing? Although testing supplies may be expensive, most insurance companies cover the cost. For uninsured patients, there are programs that assist with the costs.
- Is the patient compliant with the testing? Frequent testing can be an essential component of blood glucose control.

---

[3]From Yoost BL, Crawford LR: *Fundamentals of nursing: Active learning for collaborative practice*, St. Louis, 2016, Mosby.

CHAPTER 31

Medication Administration

MEDICATION TERMINOLOGY

Absorption: The passage of drug molecules into the blood.

Abuse: A maladaptive pattern of drug usage.

Allergic reaction: An unpredictable response to a drug.

Biotransformation: Drug metabolism from an active to an inactive state.

Classification: Indicates the effect on a body system.

Distribution: How a drug is absorbed into the body tissues.

Duration: Length of time in the body.

Excretion: The exit of the drug from the body.

Form: Determines the routes of administration.

Genetic difference: The makeup by which a person's genetic background may affect a drug's actions in the body.

Half-life: Time of elimination from body.
Idiosyncratic: Drugs that are overactive or underactive.
Interactions: When one drug modifies the actions of another.
Medication: A substance used in the treatment, cure, relief, or prevention of disease.
Onset: First response of drug in the body.
Peak: Highest level of drug in the body.
Pharmacokinetics: The study of how drugs enter the body, reach their site of action, are metabolized, and exit the body.
Physiologic variables: The normal difference between men and women and differences in weight may affect the metabolism of a drug.
Plateau: Concentration of dose levels.
Side effects: Unintended secondary effects.
Standards: Guidelines for purity and quality of a drug.
Therapeutic: Beneficial level of drug.
Tolerance: Low response to a drug.
Toxic: Not beneficial or lethal level of drug.
Trough: Lowest level of drug in the body.

Controlled Substances
Schedule I: Highest potential for abuse: heroin, LSD, marijuana
Schedule II: High potential for abuse: opioids, amphetamines, barbiturates
Schedule III: Potential for abuse: steroids, codeine, ketamine, hydrocodone
Schedule IV: Low potential for abuse: Valium, Xanax, phenobarbital
Schedule V: Lowest potential for abuse: cough suppressants

EQUIVALENT MEASURES
Metric System
To change from a larger to a smaller unit, MULTIPLY the number by 10, 100, and so on or move the decimal point to the RIGHT. To change from a smaller to larger unit, DIVIDE the number by 10, 100, and so on or move the decimal to the LEFT.

Weight
1 kilogram (kg/Kg)	=	1000 grams (g)
1 gram (Gm/gm/g/G)	=	1000 milligrams (mg)
1 milligram (mg)	=	1000 micrograms (mcg)

Volume
1 liter (L)	=	1000 milliliters (mL)
1 deciliter (dL)	=	100 milliliters (mL)
1 milliliter (mL)	=	1 cubic centimeter (cc)

Length
1 meter (m)	=	100 centimeters (cm)
1 meter (m)	=	1000 millimeters (mm)
1 centimeter (cm)	=	10 millimeters (mm)

Apothecary System
Weight: grains (gr); volume: minims (m), drams (dr), ounces (oz)

Metric-to-Apothecary Conversions
Grams to grains: Multiply grams (g) by 15
Milligrams to grains: Divide milligrams (mg) by 60

Apothecary-to-Metric Conversions
Grains to grams: Divide grains (gr) by 15
Grains to milligrams: Multiply grains (gr) by 60

Household System
Weight
1 tablespoon (tbsp/T)	=	3 teaspoons (tsp/t)
1 cup (c)	=	16 tablespoons (tbsp/T)
1 pound (lb)	=	16 ounces (oz)

Volume
1 gallon (gal)	=	4 quarts (qt)
1 quart (qt)	=	2 pints (pt)
1 pint (pt)	=	2 cups (c)
1 cup (c)	=	8 ounces (oz)
30 cc	=	1 ounce (oz)

Kilogram-to-Pound Conversions
Kilograms to pounds: Multiply kilograms (kg) by 2.2

Pounds to kilograms: Divide pounds (lb) by 2.2

Household-Metric Conversions
15 drops (gtt)	=	1 mL
1 tsp/t	=	5 mL
1 tbsp/T	=	15 mL
1 cup/c	=	240 mL
1 pint/pt	=	≈480 mL
1 quart/qt	=	≈960 mL
1 gallon/gal	=	≈3785 mL or 4 L

CALCULATING IV DRIP RATES
The *drops per 1 mL* is the number of drops needed to fill a 1-mL syringe.

The *rate* is the number of milliliters per hour.

The *drip rate* is the amount of volume divided by the time needed to infuse.

Following is the equation that can be used to
  calculate IV drip rates:
Microdrops: A Simple Calculation
10 drops or gtt: mL/hr=gtt/min per micro divided by 6
15 drops or gtt: mL/hr=gtt/min per micro divided by 4
20 drops or gtt: mL/hr=gtt/min per micro divided by 3
60 drops or gtt/mL: mL/hr=gtt/min

MEDICATION SAFETY
Ten Patient Rights
  1. Right patient
  2. Right drug
  3. Right dose
  4. Right route
  5. Right time
  6. Right assessment
  7. Right documentation
  8. Right to know
  9. Right evaluation
  10. Right to refuse

Six Rights for Safe Medication Administration[1]
1. The right to a complete written order
2. The right to a correctly dispensed medication
3. The right to have access to drug and patient
   information
4. The right to have policies on medication
   administration
5. The right to identify problems in the system
6. The right to stop, think, and be vigilant about
   medication administration

---

[1]Adapted from Cook MC: Nurses' six rights for safe medication
administration, *Mass Nurse* 69(6):8, 1999.

ASSESSMENT QUESTIONS RELATED TO MEDICATIONS[2]

- What food or drug allergies do you have? Describe the reaction.
- What prescribed medications are you currently taking? Do you have them with you?
- Which over-the-counter medications and herbs do you take on a regular basis (e.g., antacids, laxatives, aspirin, creams or lotions)?
- What is your alcohol intake? Caffeine intake? Use of home remedies?
- What medications have you stopped taking recently?
- Do you use any other methods to relieve your symptoms?
- When you feel better do you stop taking your medications? If so, which ones?
- Do you sometimes forget to take your medications? If so, under what circumstances?
- When you are traveling, do you forget to take your medications?
- What times do you take your medications?
- Do you prepare your medications in a special way (crushed in applesauce, with a meal)?
- How do you remember to take your medications on schedule?
- Have you had any side effects or adverse reactions from medications?
- Can you tell me why you take this medication?
- Are there problems that prevent you from taking your medications (e.g., cost, access at work or school, irregular meal schedules)?
- How do you feel about taking medications?

---

[2]From Yoost BL, Crawford LR: *Fundamentals of nursing: Active learning for collaborative practice,* St. Louis, 2016, Mosby.

HOME CARE RELATED TO MEDICATIONS[3]

- Discharge planning should include teaching patients, family members, and caregivers how to safely administer medications in the home.
- A medication regimen should account for lifestyle, be easy to remember, and be convenient for the patient. Assistive devices, such as a pill organizer or an automated phone reminder system, can help patients remember to take medications.
- Linking medication times with normal events in the day, such as meals or bedtime, increases accurate and continued use of medications.
- Assess for any factors that may affect the safe use of medications, such as poor memory or poor vision.
- Referrals to social services for financial assistance programs and drug company assistance programs can help address financial needs for obtaining medications.
- Medications disposed of in the trash or flushed down the toilet can leak into the water supply and contaminate it.
- Educate about proper disposal of needles.

VITAMINS AND ADVERSE EFFECTS[4]
Water-Soluble Vitamins

B_3 (niacin): Flushing, redness of the skin, upset stomach.

B_6 (pyridoxine, pyridoxal, and pyridoxamine): Nerve damage to the limbs, which may cause numbness, trouble walking, and pain.

---

[3]From Yoost BL, Crawford LR: *Fundamentals of nursing: Active learning for collaborative practice,* St. Louis, 2016, Mosby.
[4]From U.S. Food and Drug Administration: *Fortify your knowledge about vitamins,* Washington, DC, 2009, U.S. Department of Health and Human Services.

C (ascorbic acid): Upset stomach, kidney stones, increased iron absorption.

Folic acid (folate): At high levels, especially in older adults, may hide signs of B_{12} deficiency.

Fat-Soluble Vitamins

- **A (retinol, retinal, retinoic acid):** Nausea, vomiting, headache, dizziness, blurred vision, clumsiness, birth defects, liver problems, possible risk of osteoporosis.
- **D (calciferol):** Nausea, vomiting, poor appetite, constipation, weakness, weight loss, confusion, heart rhythm problems, deposits of calcium and phosphate in soft tissues.

CULTURAL FACTORS RELATED TO MEDICATIONS

- Herbal medicine used in a culture may affect the action of prescribed medications.
- Certain cultural and religious groups have beliefs that discourage the use of medications other than natural remedies.

CHAPTER 32

Perioperative Nursing Care

COMMON SURGICAL PROCEDURES

Anastomosis: Creation of a passage between two vessels.

Angiectomy or angioplasty: Removal or repair of a vessel.

Aortotomy: Incision into the aorta.

Arteriectomy or arterioplasty: Removal or repair of an artery.

Arthrectomy or arthroplasty: Removal or repair of a joint.

Atriotomy: Incision into an atrium of heart.

Biopsy: Incision to remove a tissue sample.

Bronchotomy or bronchoplasty: Incision into repair of bronchus.

Cholecystectomy: Removal of the gallbladder.

Choledochectomy: Removal of a portion of the common bile duct.

Colectomy: Partial removal of the colon.

Coronary artery bypass graft (CABG): A large vein from the body is removed and sutured to either side of an obstructed coronary artery.

Craniectomy or cranioplasty: Removal or repair of a portion of the skull.

Cystectomy or cystoplasty: Removal or repair of the bladder.

Dermabrasion: Surgical removal of epidermis or a portion of the dermis.

Embolization: Suturing or sealing of a vessel.

Esophagectomy or esophagoplasty: Removal or repair of the esophagus.

Fasciectomy or fascioplasty: Removal or repair of the fascia.

Gastrectomy or gastroplasty: Removal or repair of the stomach.

Graft: Surgical replacement of tissue, skin, or muscle.

Hysterectomy: Removal of the uterus.

Laminectomy: Removal of the posterior arch of a vertebra.

Laryngectomy or laryngoplasty: Removal or repair of the larynx.

Lymphangiectomy or lymphangioplasty: Removal or repair of a lymph vessel.

Mastectomy or mastopexy: Removal or reduction of a breast.

Myectomy or myoplasty: Removal or repair of an ovary.

Nephrectomy: Removal of a kidney.

Oophorectomy or oophoroplasty: Removal or repair of a testicle.

Orchiectomy or orchioplasty: Removal or repair of a testicle.

Osteoclasis: Reconstruction of a fractured bone.

Percutaneous transluminal coronary angioplasty (PTCA): A balloon procedure used to push an obstruction against a vessel wall to allow blood to flow through.

Pericardiectomy: Removal of the pericardium.

Phlebectomy or phleboplasty: Removal or repair of a vein.

Pneumonectomy: Removal of a lung.

Radical mastectomy: Removal of a breast, pectorals, lymph nodes, and skin.

Rhinoplasty: Plastic repair of the nose.

Splenotomy or splenorrhaphy: Incision into or repair of the spleen.

Thoracoplasty: Removal of a rib to allow collapse of the lungs.

Valvulotomy or valvuloplasty: Incision into or repair of a valve.

NURSING CARE BEFORE SURGERY

Teaching: Include the following information:

- Smoking or drinking restrictions before surgery
- Dietary or fluid restrictions before surgery
- Review of surgical procedure
- Postoperative deep breathing, positioning, and range-of-motion exercises
- Postoperative pain and pain relief measures available
- Postoperative activity or dietary restrictions
- Postoperative dressing procedures
- Review of drains, nasogastric, catheter, and intravenous (IV) lines that may be inserted during surgery

History intake: Include the following information:

- Chief complaint or reason for surgery
- Prior surgeries and responses or impressions
- Drug allergies

- Physical limitations such as vision or hearing problems, limps, or paralysis
- History of smoking and drinking
- Last drink or food intake
- Medications and the last time taken
- Nonprescription or recreational drug use and when taken last
- History of strokes, heart attacks, seizures, diabetes, and thyroid or adrenal disease
- Concerns, questions, or special requests
- Significant other and where he or she can be reached after surgery

PRESURGICAL CHECKLIST

Include the following information:

- Signed consent form in front of the chart
- List of clothes and valuables and their placement in a safe place
- Record of vital signs and last time voided
- List of prostheses such as dentures and limbs removed
- List of preoperative medications and when administered
- Review of preoperative laboratory values and tests

PREOPERATIVE SURGICAL SCRUBS

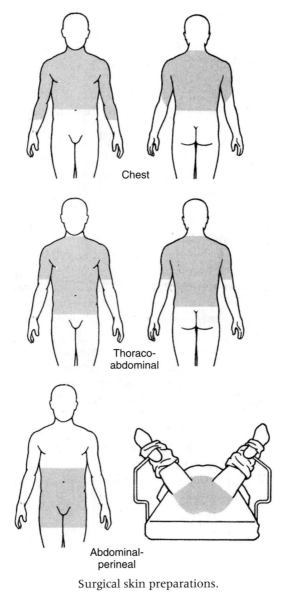

Chest

Thoraco-
abdominal

Abdominal-
perineal

Surgical skin preparations.

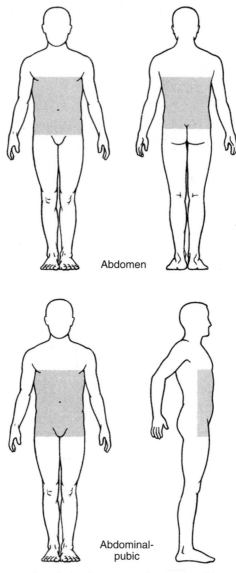

Abdomen

Abdominal-
pubic

Surgical skin preparations—cont'd.

NURSING CARE AFTER SURGERY
- Provide a safe environment for the patient
- Monitor the patient's condition
- Recognize potential complications
- Prevent complications

Information Needed
- Type of surgery and anesthetic
- Findings and results of the surgery
- Any complications during the surgery
- Estimated blood loss and if any transfusions were given during surgery
- Current respiratory condition of the patient
- Current cardiac and circulatory condition of the patient
- Types and number of incisions, drains, tubes, and IV lines
- Current vital signs and when they need to be taken next
- Current laboratory values and when specimens need to be drawn next
- Dressing location, condition, and changes (the first change is generally done by the surgeon)
- Neurologic status and need for future neurologic checks
- Time, frequency, and route of administration of pain medications
- Additional postoperative orders
- Notify any family or significant others waiting for the patient

ASSESSMENT OF BODY SYSTEMS AFTER SURGERY
Cardiac
- Possibility of hemorrhage, shock, embolism, thrombosis
- Monitor blood pressure, heart rate, rhythm, quality

- Check for Homans sign, leg tenderness, leg edema
- Check capillary refill, hemorrhage, shock, pedal pulses

Pulmonary
- Possibility of obstruction, atelectasis, pneumonia
- Turn patient every 1 to 2 hours unless contraindicated
- Have patient cough and deep breathe using pillows to splint incisions every 1 to 2 hours
- Assess lungs for rales, rhonchi, or wheezes
- Check oxygen saturation per policy protocol or with each check of vital signs
- Perform oral or deep suction as needed
- Have patient use incentive spirometer as ordered every 1 to 2 hours
- Use humidification to ease breathing and chest therapy if ordered
- Ensure adequate hydration to help thin secretions and postural drainage to drain secretions
- Assess for adequate pain relief to help breathing

Neurologic
- Perform neurologic and reflex checks as needed
- Assess orientation, level of consciousness, and pain control as needed
- Assess for restlessness, fatigue, and anxiety
- Explain the need for the procedure to the patient

Genitourinary
- Assess for adequate fluid intake and output and for bladder distention
- Assess the need for and care of Foley catheter or need for straight catheterization

Gastrointestinal
- Assess bowel sounds for possible ileus (indicated by no sounds)
- Assess for nausea, vomiting, distended abdomen, and gas pains

Skin
- Assess wound for drainage and signs of infection
- Assess for skin breakdown

COUGH AND DEEP BREATHING TECHNIQUE
- Breathing techniques used by postoperative patients:
  - Controlled cough
  - Deep breaths in through the nose and exhaled through the mouth
  - Diaphragmatic breathing and pursed-lip exhalation
- Benefits of the techniques:
  - Maintenance of lung expansion
  - Prevention of atelectasis and pneumonia

If surgery is planned, the patient will benefit most from being taught one or more of these techniques *before* surgery to allow time to practice them before they are needed.

PULMONARY EMBOLI
Venous stasis is commonly seen in postoperative patients, which creates a risk for clots to develop and a portion of a thrombus to break away from the wall of the vein and travel to the heart, lungs, or brain. Patients with this disorder often present with one or more of the following:
- Anxiety
- Chest pain

- Cough
- Cyanosis
- Dyspnea
- Arrhythmia
- Hypotension
- Leg pain and swelling (in one or both legs)
- Restlessness
- Tachycardia
- Tachypnea

TYPES OF DRESSING CHANGES

Name	Uses
Absorbent	Drains wound (increases evaporation)
Antiseptic	Prevents infection
Dry	With wound with little or no drainage
Hot and moist	Promotes wound healing by second or third intention; increases blood supply to wound
Occlusive	Prevents invasion of bacteria
Protective	Protects wound from injury
Wet to damp	Dressing removed before wound dries
Wet to dry	With open wound that has necrotic tissue; wound with greatest drainage
Wet to wet	With wound that needs to be kept very moist

CHAPTER 33

Oxygenation and Tissue Perfusion

NORMAL BREATH SOUNDS

Vesicular: Soft, low-pitched sighing over bronchiole and alveoli base on inspiration.

Bronchial: Moderate, high-pitched sound over trachea.

Bronchovesicular: Moderate sound over first and second intercostal spaces.

Tracheal: Loudest and highest pitched of normal breath sounds, harsh and tubular.

SIGNS AND SYMPTOMS OF HYPERVENTILATION, HYPOVENTILATION, AND HYPOXIA

Signs and Symptoms of Hyperventilation

- Tachycardia, chest pain, shortness of breath
- Dizziness, light-headedness, disorientation

- Paresthesia, numbness
- Tinnitus, blurred vision, tetany

Signs and Symptoms of Hypoventilation
- Dizziness, headache, lethargy
- Disorientation, convulsions, coma
- Decreased ability to follow instructions
- Cardiac arrhythmias, electrolyte imbalance, cardiac arrest

Signs and Symptoms of Hypoxia
- Restlessness, anxiety, disorientation
- Decreased concentration, fatigue
- Decreased consciousness, dizziness
- Behavioral changes, pallor
- Increased pulse and blood pressure
- Cardiac arrhythmias, cyanosis, clubbing, dyspnea

ABNORMAL AND ADVENTITIOUS SOUNDS
Crackles/rales: Fine, crackle-like sounds, usually on inspiration
- **Alveolar:** High pitched
- **Bronchial:** Low pitched

Rhonchi: Coarse, harsh, over fluid (usually on expiration)

Wheezes: Squeaky, musical on inspiration or expiration

Friction rub: Grating sound of pleurae rubbing together, generally on the anterior side

ASSESSMENT OF RESPIRATORY STATUS
Time Pattern
- When did the breathing sound start?
- How long did it last?
- Is there a pattern to the occurrences?

Quality
- How would you describe it?

Relieving Factors
- What makes it better?

Aggravating Factors
- What makes it worse?

Other
- What other symptoms are also present?
- Is there any coughing?
- Is there any difficulty breathing?

TESTS FOR ABNORMAL BREATH SOUNDS
Chest x-ray
Pulmonary function tests
Blood tests (including an arterial blood gas)
CT scan of the chest
Analysis of a sputum sample

PULMONARY FUNCTION TESTS
- **Forced vital capacity** (FVC) measures the volume of air the patient can forcefully expire after the maximum amount of air is breathed in. The normal amount is 4 L.
- **Forced expiratory volume in one second** (FEV_1) measures the volume of air expired in one second from the beginning of the FVC. The expected finding is 3.0 L or 84% of FVC.
- **Forced expiratory flow** (FEF) measures the maximal flow rate that is attained during the middle of the FVC maneuver. The expected findings vary by body size.

- **Residual volume** (RV) is the amount of air remaining in the lungs after maximum expiration. The expected finding is 1.2 L.
- **Functional residual capacity** (FRC) is the volume of air that remains in the patient's lung after normal expiration. The predicted volume is 2.3 L.

OXYGEN THERAPY

Oxygen is considered a drug; therefore a physician's order is required.

Cannula

- $1 L = 24\% \ O_2$
- $2 L = 28\% \ O_2$
- $3 L = 32\% \ O_2$
- $4 L = 36\% \ O_2$
- $5 L = 40\% \ O_2$
- $6 L = 44\% \ O_2$
- If patient requires more oxygen than 6 L of O_2, a mask may be needed.
- Humidification may be added for comfort.

Simple Mask

- 5 to $6 L = 40\%$ to $45\% \ O_2$
- 7 to $8 L = 50\%$ to $55\% \ O_2$
- 9 to $10 L = 60\% \ O_2$
- *Should not be run below 5 L/min.*

Partial Rebreathing Mask

- 6 to $10 L = $ Up to $80\% \ O_2$
- Level of O_2 will depend on patient's overall respiratory and health status.
- Should not be run below 5 L/min. Reservoir bag should never be fully collapsed.

ABNORMAL BREATHING PATTERNS

Type	Characteristics	Assess for
Apnea	Periods of not breathing	Sleep problem, impending death
Bradypnea	<10 breaths/min	Drug overdose, alcohol overdose
Dyspnea	Difficulty breathing	Low hemoglobin, acidosis
Stridor	High-pitched sounds	Obstruction
Tachypnea	>20 breaths/min	Anxiety, fever
Hyperpnea	Increased rate and depth	Pain, reaction to altitude
Hyperventilation	Increased rate and depth	Acidosis
Cheyne-Stokes breathing	Alternating periods of hyperpnea and apnea	Impending death
Kussmaul respirations	Extreme rate and depth	Diabetic ketoacidosis, renal failure
Asymmetric	Lungs do not expand equally	Fractured ribs, missing lung, pneumothorax

COMMON LUNG DISORDERS

Asthma
Signs and symptoms: Dyspnea, cough, tachypnea
Listen for: Decreased sounds with wheezes

Atelectasis
Signs and symptoms: Tachypnea, cyanosis, use of accessory muscles
Listen for: Decreased sound with crackles

Bronchiectasis
Signs and symptoms: Chronic cough with large amounts of foul-smelling sputum production, coughing up blood, cough worsened by lying on one side, fatigue, shortness of breath worsened by exercise, weight loss, wheezing, paleness, skin discoloration, bluish, breath odor; clubbing of fingers may be present
Listen for: Wheezes and crackles

Bronchitis
Signs and symptoms: Cough with sputum, sore throat and fever, prolonged expiration
Listen for: Prolonged expiration, wheezes, crackles

Cystic Fibrosis (CF)
Signs and symptoms: Recurrent respiratory infections, such as pneumonia or sinusitis; coughing or wheezing; no bowel movements in first 24 to 48 hours of life; and stools that are pale or clay colored, foul-smelling, or that float. Infants may have salty-tasting skin, weight loss, or failure to gain weight normally in childhood; diarrhea; delayed growth; and fatigue
Listen for: Wheezes and crackles

Emphysema
Signs and symptoms: Dyspnea, cough with sputum
Listen for: Wheezes, rhonchi

Interstitial Lung Disease (ILD)
Signs and symptoms: Shortness of breath during exercise; when the disease is severe and prolonged, heart failure with swelling of the legs may occur
Listen for: Dry cough without sputum

Neoplasm
Signs and symptoms: Cough with sputum, chest pain
Listen for: Decreased sounds

Pleural Effusion
Signs and symptoms: Pain, dyspnea, pallor, fever, cough
Listen for: Decreased sounds, friction rub

Pneumonia
Signs and symptoms: Chills, productive cough, rapid swallow rate
Listen for: Fine crackles or friction rub

Pneumothorax
Signs and symptoms: Pain, dyspnea, cyanosis, tachypnea
Listen for: Decreased sound on affected side

Pulmonary Edema
Signs and symptoms: Tachypnea, cough, cyanosis, orthopnea, use of accessory muscles
Listen for: Rales, rhonchi, wheezes

ASSESSMENT QUESTIONS RELATED TO OXYGEN THERAPY[1]

Cardiovascular Focus

- Are you having any chest pain? If so, rate it on a scale of 0 to 10.
- How long have you had the pain?
- Is the pain located in one area or does it radiate to other areas?
- Do any activities or medications make it worse or better?
- Are any symptoms such as shortness of breath or sweating associated with the pain?
- Do you have increased fatigue?
- Have you had any recent weight gain?
- Have you had any changes in skin texture, color, or temperature?
- Do you take medications that prevent blood clots?
- Have you had any sores on your lower extremities that have not healed?
- Have you had any episodes of dizziness or loss of consciousness?
- Do you have any other chronic diseases?

Pulmonary Focus

- Have you had any times of breathing difficulties when you are exercising or at rest?
- Have you had a loss of appetite, weight loss, or weakness?
- Have you ever smoked?
- If so, are you still smoking or did you quit smoking?
- Do you sleep on one or more pillows?
- How much do you exercise?
- Do you have wheezing, pain with breathing, or difficulty clearing your secretions?

---

[1]From Yoost BL, Crawford LR: *Fundamentals of nursing: Active learning for collaborative practice,* St. Louis, 2016, Mosby.

- Have you had asthma, bronchitis, or other lung diseases in the past?
- Do you use oxygen at home?
- What type of work have you done, and were you exposed to hazardous materials?
- Do you have anxiety related to your breathing condition?
- Do you have a cough? For how long?
- Are you coughing anything up? Color of sputum?
- Is it worse when you lay down?

HOME CARE RELATED TO BREATHING[2]

- To place oxygen in a home, an order is obtained from a primary care provider; the order should have the diagnosis of a medical condition that confirms the need for home oxygen.
- A patient who is using oxygen at home must be educated on proper use and storage of oxygen.
- Signs stating "No smoking" need to be in place in the home.
- The size and configuration of the home is used to determine placement of oxygen and length of tubing to allow the patient to go from one room to another.

COMPONENTS OF A SMOKING CESSATION PROGRAM[3]

- Education about the dangers of smoking and health benefits of smoking cessation.
- Self-help materials and information on nicotine replacements.

---

[2]From Yoost BL, Crawford LR: *Fundamentals of nursing: Active learning for collaborative practice,* St. Louis, 2016, Mosby.
[3]From National Cancer Institute: Free help to quit smoking, n.d. Retrieved from *www.cancer.gov/cancertopics/tobacco/smoking.*

- Being aware of smoking triggers and planning ways to cope with them.
- Counseling and support in person or by telephone and alternative therapy approaches.
- Use of problem-solving approach such as planning a day without smoking.
- Non-nicotine medications (bupropion) work on parts of the brain that are involved with nicotine addiction.

CHAPTER 34

Fluid, Electrolyte, and Acid-Base Balance

FLUID VOLUME DEFICIT
Fluid volume deficit occurs with excessive loss or inadequate intake of fluid. Two types of fluid deficits can occur: isotonic (hypovolemia) and hypertonic **(dehydration)**.

Hypovolemia
Signs and symptoms: Hypotension, weight loss, decreased tearing or saliva, dry skin or mouth, oliguria, increased pulse or respirations, increased specific gravity of urine, increased serum sodium levels.

Causes: Dehydration, insufficient fluid intake, diuretics, sweating or polyuria, excessive tube feedings leading to diarrhea.
- 2% loss of total body weight (TBW) is mild dehydration
- 5% loss of TBW is moderate dehydration
- 8% loss of TBW is severe dehydration
- 15% loss of TBW is life threatening, usually fatal

FLUID VOLUME EXCESS
Fluid volume excess occurs when fluid intake exceeds output. Severity of the fluid volume excess is assessed by the corresponding increase in TBW.

Hypervolemia
Signs and symptoms: Edema, puffy face or eyelids, ascites, rales or wheezes in lungs, bounding pulse, hypertension, sudden weight gain, decreased serum sodium levels.
Causes: Overhydration, renal failure, congestive heart failure.
- 2% gain of TBW is mild excess
- 5% gain of TBW is moderate excess
- 8% gain of TBW is severe excess

EDEMA GRADING SCALE
1+ Barely detectable
2+ Indentation of less than 5 mm
3+ Indentation of 5 to 10 mm
4+ Indentation of greater than 10 mm

AVERAGE DAILY FLUID INTAKE AND OUTPUT

Intake (mL)		Output (mL)	
Fluids	1600	Urine	1500
Food	700	Feces	200
Metabolism	200	Skin (including perspiration)	500
		Lungs	300
Total Intake	2500	*Total Output*	2500

From Yoost BL, Crawford LR: *Fundamentals of nursing: Active learning for collaborative practice,* St. Louis, 2016, Mosby.

COMMON INTRAVENOUS SOLUTIONS
Hypotonic
Normal saline (NS) 0.33%: Provides sodium, chloride, and free water. Allows kidneys to select amount of electrolyte to retain or excrete.

Normal saline (NS) 0.45%: Useful for determining renal function. Not used as replacement therapy.

Isotonic
D_5W: Considered isotonic but becomes free water after dextrose is metabolized; will act as a hypotonic solution. Because it does not contain sodium, continued use can lead to hyponatremia. Useful in IV medication administration.

Normal saline (NS) 0.9%: Commonly used to reestablish normal extracellular fluid levels in patients with hypovolemia. Not used as a maintenance fluid; continued use can lead to hypernatremia.

D$_5$ 0.2% NS: Useful for maintenance of fluids when less sodium is required. The dextrose provides approximately 170 calories per liter.

Lactated Ringer's (LR): Most resembles blood plasma. Contains sodium, potassium, calcium, chloride, and lactate. Used when there is loss of both fluid and electrolytes as in burns or severe diarrhea.

Hypertonic

D$_5$ 0.45% NS: Commonly used to treat hypovolemia and maintain normal fluid balance.

D$_5$ 0.9% NS: Used as replacement fluid. Will provide calories, sodium, and chloride. Prolonged use can lead to hypernatremia.

D$_5$ LR: Same content as Lactated Ringer's but adds calories with the dextrose. Useful when patient's caloric intake is reduced.

3% NS: Used to treat severe hyponatremia. Administered in an intensive care setting where the patient can be closely monitored.

RED BLOOD CELL TRANSFUSION

- **Typing:** Selecting the ABO blood type and Rh antigen factor of a person's blood (other antigens can also affect transfusion compatibility).
- **Cross-matching:** Mixing the recipient's serum with the donor's red blood cells in a saline solution; if no agglutination occurs, the blood may be safely given.

Before Administering Blood to a Patient

- Check facility's policy on infusing blood products.
- Check the patient's ID band for proper identification.
- Check the patient's blood type and Rh antigen.
- Get the blood from blood bank only when ready to infuse.
- Compare the patient's blood type with the type of blood to be infused.
- Two people should check and cosign blood.

- Start infusion of blood with normal saline solution.
- Administer blood at a slower rate for the first 15 minutes. Blood should be infused within 4 hours.
- Use appropriate blood tubing and needles (may vary per facility).
- Document action on appropriate flow sheets (may vary per facility).
- Instruct patient to report *any* discomfort (blood reactions).
- Special vital signs are needed (may vary per facility).
- Some facilities may medicate the patient with acetaminophen or diphenhydramine (Benadryl) before infusion.

Blood Reactions
- Possible reactions include difficulty breathing, wheezing, tachypnea, fever, tachycardia, change in blood pressure, chest pain, disorientation, rash, or hives.
- *If a reaction begins, stop the infusion.* Begin a normal saline flush to keep the IV line open and administer prescribed antihistamines.

Blood Type Compatibility		
Blood Type	**Can Generally Donate to**	**Can Generally Receive From**
A–	A–, A+	A–, O–
B–	B–, B+	B–, O–
AB–	AB–, AB+	AB–, A–, B–, O
A+	A+	A+, A–, O+, O–
B+	B+	B+, B–, O+, O–
AB+	AB+	All blood types
O–	All blood types	O–
O+	O+, A+, B+, AB+	O+, O–

- Notify a physician, recheck blood, retype, and cross-match. Do *not* discard the blood—the laboratory may want to analyze it for the cause of the reaction. The physician may require a urine sample from the patient.

ELECTROLYTE IMBALANCES
Hyponatremia (less than 135 mEq/L)
Signs and symptoms: Fatigue; abdominal cramps; diarrhea; weakness; hypotension; cool, clammy skin.

Causes: Overhydration, kidney disease, diarrhea, syndrome of inappropriate antidiuretic hormone secretion (SIADH).

Hypernatremia (greater than 145 mEq/L)
Signs and symptoms: Thirst; dry, sticky mucous membranes; dry tongue and skin; flushed skin; increased body temperature.

Causes: Dehydration, starvation.

Hypokalemia (less than 3.5 mEq/L)
Signs and symptoms: Weakness, fatigue, anorexia, abdominal distention, arrhythmias, decreased bowel sounds.

Causes: Diarrhea, diuretics, alkalosis, polyuria.

Hyperkalemia (greater than 5 mEq/L)
Signs and symptoms: Anxiety, arrhythmias, increased bowel sounds.

Causes: Burns, renal failure, dehydration, acidosis.

Hypocalcemia (less than 8.3 mEq/L)
Signs and symptoms: Abdominal cramps, tingling, muscle spasms, convulsions; assess magnesium level.

Causes: Parathyroid dysfunction, vitamin D deficiency, pancreatitis.

Hypercalcemia (greater than 10 mEq/L)
Signs and symptoms: Deep bone pain, nausea, vomiting, constipation; assess magnesium level.
Causes: Parathyroid tumor, bone cancer or metastasis, osteoporosis.

Hypomagnesemia (less than 1.3 mEq/L)
Signs and symptoms: Tremors, muscle cramps, tachycardia, hypertension, confusion; assess calcium level.
Causes: Parathyroid dysfunction, cancer, chemotherapy, polyuria.

Hypermagnesemia (greater than 2.5 mEq/L)
Signs and symptoms: Lethargy, respiratory difficulty, coma; assess calcium level.
Causes: Parathyroid dysfunction, renal failure.

Hypochloremia (less than 96 mEq/L)
Signs and symptoms: Fatigue, weakness, dizziness.
Causes: Loss of fluid, severe vomiting or diarrhea, prolonged diuretic or laxative use.

Hyperchloremia (greater than 108 mEq/L)
Signs and symptoms: Thirst; dry mucous membranes, tongue, and skin.
Causes: High sodium level, kidney failure, diabetes insipidus, diabetic coma.

Hypophosphatemia (less than 2.2 mEq/L)
Signs and symptoms: Nausea, bone and joint pain, constipation.
Causes: After stomach surgery, lack of vitamin D, high calcium levels, kidney damage, several endocrine disorders.

Hyperphosphatemia (greater than 4.8 mEq/L)
Signs and symptoms: Abdominal cramps, numbness and tingling.
Causes: Excess dairy intake, increased vitamin D, low calcium levels, kidney failure, tumor lysis syndrome.

ARTERIAL BLOOD GAS RESULTS WITH ACID–BASE IMBALANCES

Acid-Base Imbalance	pH	PaCO$_2$	HCO$_3$
Respiratory acidosis	↓	↑	Normal
Respiratory alkalosis	↑	↓	Normal
Metabolic acidosis	↓	Normal	↓
Metabolic alkalosis	↑	Normal	↑

ACID–BASE IMBALANCES
Respiratory Acidosis
Underlying causes: Chest or brainstem injury, asthma attack, pulmonary edema.
Medications: Anesthetics, opioids, sedatives.
Clinical manifestations: Headache, altered consciousness, irritability, confusion, dyspnea, tachycardia, muscle twitching.
- Uncompensated ABG results: pH <7.45, HCO$_3$ normal.
- Partially compensated ABG results: pH <7.45, HCO$_3$ >26 mEq.
- As compensation continues, the pH will increase.
Nursing interventions: Assess vital signs, especially rate and depth of respirations, pulse oximetry. Assess breath sounds and cardiac rhythm, administer oxygen as ordered. Monitor

ABG results. Have mechanical ventilation available. Encourage deep breathing and coughing. Encourage fluid intake.

Respiratory Alkalosis

Underlying causes: Pain, hyperventilation, salicylate or nicotine overdose, increased metabolic states.

Clinical manifestations: Tachypnea (rapid, shallow breathing), numbness, tingling of fingers, muscle cramping, palpitations, anxiety, restlessness, ECG changes.

- ABG results: pH > 7.45, $PaCO_2$ < 35 mm Hg, HCO_3 normal; will fall < 22 mEq if the imbalance is compensated.

Nursing interventions: Assess vital signs. Encourage patient if tachypneic to take slow, deep breaths. Monitor ABGs, provide reassurance to anxious patient.

Metabolic Acidosis

Underlying causes: Shock, trauma, cardiac arrest, diabetic ketoacidosis, chronic renal failure, salicylate, overdose, sepsis, chronic diarrhea.

Clinical manifestations: Kussmaul respirations, hypotension, headache, decreased level of consciousness, weakness, nausea, vomiting, anorexia.

- ABG results pH < 7.35, $PaCO_2$ normal; will fall < 35 mm Hg if the imbalance is compensated HCO_3 < 22 mEq.

Nursing interventions: Assess vital signs, especially respiratory rate and rhythm, blood pressure, and pulse oximetry. Monitor cardiac rhythm and ABGs and serum electrolytes, glucose, BUN/creatinine. Monitor level of consciousness, have mechanical ventilation available as needed, administer sodium bicarbonate as ordered.

Metabolic Alkalosis

Underlying causes: Vomiting, nasogastric suctioning. Overuse of bicarbonate antacids, hypokalemia, loop and thiazide diuretics.

Clinical manifestations: Hypotension, mental confusion, muscle twitching, tetany, increased deep tendon reflexes, numbness, tingling of fingers and toes, seizures. Anorexia, nausea, vomiting, polyuria.

- ABG results: pH > 7.45, $PaCO_2$ normal; will rise > 45 mm Hg if the imbalance is compensated HCO_3 > 26 mEq.

Nursing interventions: Assess vital signs, especially cardiac rate and rhythm, respiration rate and depth, pulse oximetry, blood pressure; monitor ABGs and serum electrolytes, especially potassium; assess level of consciousness, administer oxygen as ordered, seizure precautions, and treat hypokalemia if appropriate.

CHAPTER 35

Bowel Elimination

FECAL CHARACTERISTICS

Characteristic	Normal	Abnormal	Assess for
Color	Brown	Clay or white	Bile obstruction
		Black or tarry	Upper GI bleeding, iron
		Red	Lower GI bleeding, beets
		Pale	Malabsorption of fat
		Green	Infection
Consistency	Moist	Hard	Constipation, dehydration
	Formed	Loose	Diet, diarrhea, medications
		Watery	Infection
		Liquid	Impaction
Odor	Aromatic	Pungent	Infection, blood
Frequency	1-2 times per day	5 times per day	Infection, diet
	Once every 3 days	Once every 6 days	Constipation, activity, medications
Shape	Cylindric	Narrow, "ribbon-like"	Obstruction

ALTERED BOWEL ELIMINATION PATTERNS

Constipation

Presence of large quantity of dry, hard feces that is difficult to expel; frequency of bowel movements is not a factor.

Causes: Reabsorption of too much water in the lower bowel as a result of medication such as narcotics, ignoring the urge to defecate, immobility, chronic laxative abuse, low fluid intake, low fiber intake, aging, postoperative conditions, or pregnancy.

Remedies: Increase fluids, fiber cereals, fruits and vegetables, exercise, and avoid cheese.

Impaction

Hard, dry stool embedded in rectal folds; may have liquid stool passing around impaction.

Causes: Poor bowel habits, immobility, inadequate food or fluids, or barium in rectum.

Remedies: Digitally remove impaction, increase fluids and fiber, increase exercise, and institute bowel program.

Diarrhea

Expulsion of fecal matter that contains too much water.

Causes: Infection, anxiety, stress, medications, too many laxatives at one time, or food or drug allergies or reactions.

Remedies: Add bulk or fiber to diet, maintain fluids and electrolytes, eat smaller amounts of food at one time, add cheese or bananas to diet, and rest after eating.

Incontinence

Inability to hold feces in rectum because of impairment of sphincter control.

Causes: Surgery, cancer, radiation treatment of rectum, paralysis, or aging.

Remedies: Bowel training, regular meal times, regular elimination patterns.

Abdominal Distention

Tympanites, or enlargement of the abdomen with gas or air as a result of excessive swallowing of air, eating gas-producing foods, or an inability to expel gas.

Causes: Constipation, fecal impaction, or postoperative conditions.

Remedies: Rectal tube can be used to expel air; increase ambulation, and change position in bed.

Obstruction

Occurs when the lumen of the bowel narrows or closes completely.

Causes: External compression can be caused by tumor; internal narrowing can be caused by impacted feces.

Remedies: Remove impaction or tumor.

Ileus (Paralytic Ileus)

Occurs when the bowel has decreased motility.

Causes: Surgery, long-term narcotic use, or complete obstruction.

Remedies: Medical intervention for physical obstructions. Specific action depend on the cause of the ileus.

FOODS THAT AFFECT BOWEL ELIMINATION PATTERNS

The following foods thicken stool:
- Bananas, rice, bread, potatoes
- Creamy peanut butter, applesauce
- Cheese, yogurt, pasta, pretzels
- Tapioca, marshmallows

The following foods loosen stool:
- Chocolate, raw fruits and vegetables
- Spiced foods, greasy or fried foods
- Prunes, grapes, leafy green vegetables

The following foods should be avoided to decrease gas:
- Beans, beer, sodas
- Cucumbers, cabbage, onions, spinach
- Brussels sprouts, broccoli, cauliflower
- Most dairy products, corn, radishes

TYPES OF CATHARTICS
- **Bulk forming:** Increases fluids and bulk in the intestines, which stimulates peristalsis. An increase in fluid is needed. *Example:* Metamucil.
- **Emollient:** Softens and delays drying of stool. *Example:* Liquid petrolatum.
- **Irritant:** Stimulates peristalsis by irritating bowel mucosa and decreasing water absorption. *Example:* Castor oil.
- **Moistening (stool softeners):** Increase water in the bowel. *Example:* Colace.
- **Saline:** When salt is in the bowel, the water will remain in the bowel as well. (Avoid use in patients with impaired renal function.) *Examples:* Milk of magnesia (MOM), Epsom salts.
- **Suppository:** Stimulates bowel and softens stool.

BENEFITS OF FIBER
- Normalization of bowel movements
- Maintenance of bowel integrity and health
- Lowering blood cholesterol levels
- Helping control blood sugar levels
- Aiding weight loss
- Potentially helping to prevent colorectal cancer

ANTIDIARRHEAL MEDICATIONS
Absorbent: Absorbs gas
Astringent: Shrinks inflamed tissues
Demulcent: Coats and protects bowel

TYPES OF ENEMAS
Carminative: Used to expel flatus
Cleansing: Stimulates peristalsis; irritates bowel by distention (use 1 L of fluid; have patient hold it as long as possible)
Colonic irrigation: Used to expel flatus
Hypertonic: Phosphates irritate bowel and draw fluid into bowel through osmosis (90 to 120 mL; hold for 10 to 15 minutes)
Hypotonic: Tap water (1 L; hold for 15 min); avoid with patients who have cardiac problems
Medicated: Contains a therapeutic agent (e.g., Kayexalate to treat high potassium levels)
Retention: Oil given to soften stool (hold for 1 hour)
Saline: Draws fluid into the bowel (9 mL of sodium to 1 L of water; hold for 15 minutes)
Soapsuds: Irritates and distends bowel (5 mL of soap to 1 L of water; hold for 15 minutes); use only Castile soaps

TYPES OF OSTOMIES
Ileostomy
Effluent: A continuous discharge that is soft and wet. The output is somewhat odorous and contains intestinal enzymes that are irritating to peristomal skin.
Skin barrier option: Highly desirable for peristomal skin protection.
Pouch option: Pouch necessary at all times.
Type of pouch: Drainable or closed-end for specific needs.
Need for irrigation: None.

Transverse Colostomy

Effluent: Usually semiliquid or very soft. Occasionally, transverse colostomy discharge is firm. Output is usually malodorous and can irritate peristomal skin. Double-barreled colostomies have two openings. Loop colostomies have one opening but two tracks—the active (proximal), which discharges fecal matter, and the inactive (distal), which discharges mucus.

Skin barrier option: Highly desirable for peristomal skin protection.

Pouch option: Pouch necessary at all times.

Type of pouch: Drainable or closed end for specific needs.

Need for irrigation: None.

Descending Colostomy or Sigmoid Colostomy

Effluent: Semisolid from descending colostomy. Firm from sigmoid colostomy. On discharge, there is an odor. Discharge is irritating if left in contact with skin around stoma. Frequency of output is unpredictable and varies with each person.

Skin barrier option: May be used for peristomal skin protection if pouch is worn.

Pouch option: Pouch should be worn if person does not irrigate.

Type of pouch: Drainable, closed end, or stoma cap.

Need for irrigation: Yes, as instructed by enterostomal (ET) nurse or physician.

Urinary Diversion (Ileal Loop, Ileal, or Colonic Conduit)

Effluent: Urine only. Output is constant. Mucus is expelled with urine. Mild odor unless there is a urinary tract infection. Urine is irritating when in contact with skin. Segment of ileum or colon is used to construct stoma.

Skin barrier option: Highly desirable for peristomal skin protection.

Pouch option: Pouch necessary at all times.
Type of pouch: Drainable pouch with spout.
Need for irrigation: None.

Continent Ileostomy

Effluent: Fluid bowel secretions are collected in a reservoir surgically constructed out of the lower part of the small intestine. Gas and feces are emptied via a surgically created leak-free nipple valve through which a catheter is inserted into the reservoir. For maximum efficiency and comfort, the reservoir is usually emptied four or five times daily. Daily schedule for catheterization should be recommended by the ET nurse or physician.

Skin barrier option: None; an absorbent pad provides peristomal skin protection.

Pouch option: None, but catheter should be available at all times.

Type of pouch: None; a drainable pouch can be applied if there is leakage of stool between intubations.

Need for irrigation: Occasionally to liquefy thick fecal matter, the pouch can be irrigated with 1 to 1.5 oz of saline or water. Specific care should be clarified by the ET nurse or physician.

Continent Urostomy

Effluent: Urine is maintained in a surgically constructed ileal pouch until emptied by means of a catheter inserted into the stoma. Uses two nipple valves—one to prevent the reflux of urine from backing up into the kidneys and the other to keep urine in the pouch until eliminated. Pouch is drained approximately four times daily. Daily schedule for pouch catheterization should be recommended by the ET nurse or physician.

Skin barrier option: None; an absorbent pad provides peristomal skin protection.

Pouch option: None, but a catheter should be available at all times.

Type of pouch: None; a urostomy pouch can be applied if there is leakage of urine between intubations.

Need for irrigation: Irrigate daily with 1 to 1.5 oz of saline solution and repeat several times as needed until the returns are clear. Specific care should be clarified by the ET nurse or physician.

CULTURAL FACTORS RELATED TO BOWEL ELIMINATION[1]

- African Americans have the highest incidence of colon cancer in the United States.
- Jews of Eastern European descent have a high risk for colorectal cancer.
- African Americans have a high incidence of lactose intolerance; it is important to check for family history.
- Dietary habits may affect bowel elimination habits and patterns.
- Cultural factors, such as the gender of the caregiver, may affect care specifically related to ostomy care.

DISABILITY FACTORS RELATED TO BOWEL ELIMINATION[2]

- Patients with physical limitations and mobility problems may have difficulty with constipation and incontinence.

[1,2]From Yoost BL, Crawford LR: *Fundamentals of nursing: Active learning for collaborative practice,* St. Louis, 2016, Mosby.

- Patients with impaired mobility may have difficulty getting to the bathroom and may need assistive devices such as bars, raised toilet seats, or elevated commodes
- Cognitive impairment such as Alzheimer disease may decrease the ability to respond to urge, contributing to constipation or incontinence.
- Patients with mental limitations may have difficulty recognizing or responding to urge.
- A slowing of nerve impulses to the anal region leads individuals to become less aware of the need to defecate, and they may develop irregular bowel movements.
- A reduction in activity levels and muscle weakness decreases peristalsis, and esophageal emptying slows.

ASSESSMENT QUESTIONS RELATED TO BOWEL ELIMINATION[3]

- Describe your daily diet and fluid intake and any recent changes.
- Describe your bowel habits and any recent changes.
- Describe the color and consistency of your stool.
- Have you been taking any medication that would cause changes in the consistency of the stool, such as laxatives, cathartics, or antibiotics?
- Have you experienced feelings of bloating or gas?
- Do you use antacid medications? If so how often? Do you notice a positive response to the medication?
- Do you have nausea or vomiting? If so, what is the onset of the nausea or vomiting? Is it related

---

[3]From Yoost BL, Crawford LR: *Fundamentals of nursing: Active learning for collaborative practice*, St. Louis, 2016, Mosby.

to particular stimuli? Are you using any types of home remedies?
- Are you experiencing any abdominal pain? If so, rate the pain on a scale of 0 to 10.
- Describe your current stress level.
- Do you work with any chemical irritants?
- Have your traveled recently? Where have you traveled?
- Have you ever been diagnosed with an abdominal disease such as cholecystitis, ulcers, diverticulitis, cholelithiasis, or cirrhosis?
- Have you had any abdominal surgery or trauma?

HOME CARE RELATED TO BOWEL FUNCTION[4]

- Family and significant others are included in ostomy teaching as this may facilitate the patient's readiness to learn.
- If the patient is apprehensive about touching or looking at the stoma, start slowly and encourage the patient's participation in care.
- Patients are given a teaching manual with step-by-step instructions, complete with illustrations, and supplemented with DVDs and access to websites.
- Evaluate the patient's home toileting facilities; note the location and availability.
- If the patient consumes gas-producing foods it may be necessary to manually expel (burp) trapped air from the bag.
  - In a private setting, the patient can undo the clasp on the flap of the bag and allow the air to be released from the bag.

---

[4]From Yoost BL, Crawford LR: *Fundamentals of nursing: Active learning for collaborative practice,* St. Louis, 2016, Mosby.

- Foods that tend to form gas, such as most beans, beer, broccoli, brussels sprouts, cabbage, carbonated beverages, eggs, fish, garlic, onions, some spices, and deep-fried or fatty foods, may be limited or avoided to help control gas and odors.
- Many products are created with an odor barrier film so that odor is contained within the pouch. Commercial deodorizing discs are available.
- Limiting odor-producing foods and emptying the pouch regularly can help reduce odor.
- Some ostomy products have a filter to allow air but not odors to escape from the pouch.

CHAPTER 36

Urinary Elimination

URINE CHARACTERISTICS

Characteristics	Normal	Abnormal	Assess for
Amount in 24 hr	1200 mL	<1200 mL	Renal failure
	1500 mL	>1500 mL	Fluid intake
Color	Straw	Amber	Dehydration, fluid intake
		Light straw	Overhydration
		Orange	Medications
		Red	Blood, injury, medications
Consistency	Clear	Cloudy, thick	Infection
Odor	Faint	Offensive	Infection, medications

	Sterile	Yes	Organisms	Infection, poor hygiene
pH		4.5	<4.5	Infection
		8.0	>8.0	Diabetes, starvation, dehydration
Specific gravity		1.010	<1.010	Diabetes insipidus, kidney failure
		1.025	>1.025	Diabetes, underhydration
Glucose		None	Present	Diabetes
Ketones		None	Present	Diabetes, starvation, vomiting
Blood		None	Present	Tumors, injury, kidney disease

ALTERED URINARY PATTERNS

Pattern	Description	Assess for
Anuria	No urination	Renal failure, dehydration, obstruction
Dysuria	Painful urination	Infection, injury, frequency, blood
Frequency	Voiding small amounts	Infection, injury, pregnancy, stress, intake
Incontinence	Difficulty with control	Infection, injury, distended bladder
Nocturia	Urinating at night	Infection, injury, pregnancy, stress, intake
Oliguria	Little urination	Infection, injury, BUN, dehydration, kidney, disease
Polyuria	Increased urination	Infection, injury, alcohol, diabetes, caffeine, diuretics, increased thirst, dehydration
Retention	Holding on to urine No urination	Infection, injury, pain, distended bladder, medications, restlessness, surgical, complications
Residual	Urine remaining in bladder after voiding	Infection, distention, pain, injury
Urgency	Urgent and immediate need to void	Infection

URINARY INCONTINENCE

Type	Description	Causes	Symptoms
Function	Involuntary and unpredictable with intact urinary and nervous systems	Changes in environment or cognitive deficits	Urge to void that causes loss of urine
Reflex	Involuntary and occurring at predictable intervals	Anesthesia, medications, spinal cord dysfunction	Lack of urge to void
Stress	Intra abdominal pressure causes leakage	Coughing, laughing, obesity, pregnancy, weak muscles	Urgency and frequency
Urge	Involuntary passage of urine with strong urgency	Small bladder capacity, bladder irritation, alcohol, caffeine	Bladder spasms, urgency and frequency
Total	Uncontrolled and continuous loss of urine	Neuropathy, trauma, fistula between bladder and vagina	Constant flow, nocturia, unaware of incontinence

REASONS FOR URINARY CATHETERS
Intermittent
- Relieve bladder distention
- Obtain a sterile specimen
- Assessment of residual urine
- Long-term management of patients with spinal cord injuries and disorders

Short-Term Indwelling
- After surgery
- Prevention of urethral obstruction
- Measurement of output in bedridden patients
- Bladder irrigation

Long-Term Indwelling
- Severe urinary retention
- Avoidance of skin rashes or infections

PREVENTION OF URINARY INFECTIONS
- Use good handwashing techniques before handling.
- Avoid raising the drainage bag above the bladder.
- Allow urine to drain freely into the bag.
- Perform good perineal care on the patient.
- Secure the catheter per procedure.
- Empty the drainage bag at least every 8 hours.
- Avoid kinking the tubing.
- Clean the spigot thoroughly before and after use.
- Avoid dragging the drainage bag on the floor.

TYPES OF URINARY CATHETERS

Type	Size
Single lumen	8-18 Fr*
Double lumen	
With inflated balloon	8-10 Fr with 3-mL balloon
	12-30 Fr with 5- to 30-mL balloon
Common male sizes	16-18 Fr
Common female sizes	12-16 Fr

Note: Triple lumen is used for continuous bladder irrigation. Coudé-tip catheter is used for men with an enlarged prostate gland.
*Fr, French.

MEDICATIONS THAT MAY DISCOLOR URINE
Dark Yellow
- Vitamin B$_2$

Orange
- Sulfonamide
- Phenazopyridine HCl (Pyridium)
- Warfarin (Coumadin)

Pink or Red
- Thorazine
- Ex-Lax
- Phenytoin (Dilantin)

Green or Blue
- Amitriptyline

Methylene Blue
- Triamterene (Dyrenium)

Brown or Black
- Iron
- Levodopa
- Nitrofurantoin
- Metronidazole (Flagyl)

LABORATORY TESTS RELATED TO URINARY ELIMINATION

Blood Urea Nitrogen
- **Reason for test:** Used to evaluate renal function.
- **Normal levels:** 7 to 20 mg/dL.
- **Abnormal levels:** Elevated levels may indicate kidney injury or disease; diabetes, high blood pressure, blockage, severe burns, gastrointestinal bleeding, dehydration or heart failure. Medications may also elevate BUN levels. Low BUN values may be caused by a low protein diet, malnutrition, liver damage, or drinking excessive amounts of liquids.

Creatinine
- **Reason for test:** Used to evaluate renal function.
- **Normal levels:** 0.6 to 1.2 mg/dL for women and 0.8 to 1.4 mg/dL for men.
- **Abnormal levels:** Patient with kidney damage will have decreased urinary creatinine but increased serum levels.

Urinalysis
Reason for test: A screening tool for UTI, kidney disease, and other conditions. Single samples can be used to determine amounts of substances such as bacteria, glucose, white blood cells, red blood cells, or proteins.

Specific Gravity
Reason for test: Monitors the balance of water and solutes (solid matter) in urine.
Abnormal levels: Specific gravity associated with dehydration is high.

pH
Reason for test: Useful in determining the kidneys' response to acid-base imbalances.
Normal levels: Urine is normally slightly acidic, with an average pH of 6. Urine with a pH of 4 is very acidic. A pH of 7 is neutral, and a pH of 9 is very alkaline.
Abnormal levels: In metabolic acidosis, the urine pH decreases as the kidneys excrete hydrogen ions; in metabolic alkalosis, pH of the urine increases. Maintaining a healthy pH helps prevent formation of kidney stones.

Protein
Reason for test: Used to determine kidney disease.
Normal levels: Normally urine does not contain protein.
Abnormal levels: Associated with fever, hard exercise, pregnancy, and kidney disease.

Glucose
Reason for test: Used to determine kidney disease or diabetes.
Normal levels: Normally urine contains little or no glucose.
Abnormal levels: Glucose in the urine may be a sign of kidney damage or disease or diabetes.

Ketones
Reason for test: Indicates that fat has been broken down for energy.

Normal levels: Ketones are normally not passed in the urine.

Abnormal levels: Large amounts of ketones in the urine may indicate diabetic ketoacidosis.

TIMED URINE TESTS

Quantitative albumin: (24 hr) Determines albumin lost in urine as a result of kidney disease, hypertension, or heart failure.

Amino acid: (24 hr) Determines the presence of congenital kidney disease.

Amylase: (2, 12, and 24 hr) Determines the presence of disease of the pancreas.

Chloride: (24 hr) Determines loss of chloride in cardiac patients on low-salt or no-salt diets.

Concentration and dilution: Determines the presence of diseases of the kidney tubules.

Creatinine clearance: (12 and 24 hr) Determines the ability of the kidneys to clear creatinine.

Estriol: (24 hr) Measures this hormone in women with high-risk pregnancies who have diabetes.

Glucose tolerance: (12 and 24 hr) Determines malfunctions of the liver and pancreas.

17-Hydroxycorticosteroid: (24 hr) Determines functioning ability of the adrenal cortex.

Urinalysis: (random times) Determines levels of bacteria, white blood cell count, red blood cell count, pH, specific gravity, protein, and bilirubin.

Urine culture: (random times) Determines the amount and type of bacteria in the urine.

Urine sensitivity: (random times) Determines the antibiotics to which the microorganisms will be sensitive or resistant.

Urobilinogen: (random times) Determines the presence of obstruction of the biliary tract.

ASSESSMENT QUESTIONS RELATED TO URINARY ELIMINATION[1]

- Have you experienced changes in your normal urination pattern? For how long?
- Have you noticed any changes in the quality, quantity, color, or odor of the urine? For how long?
- Are you able to control when you urinate?
- Do you have difficulty starting or stopping your flow of urine?
- Have you noticed difficulty initiating the stream of urine? Voiding in small amounts?
- Do you ever have to get up at night to urinate?
- Have you ever been diagnosed with kidney or bladder disease?
- Have you ever had surgery or experienced trauma to the urinary system?
- Have you ever had a urinary tract or kidney infection?
- Do you have a family history of kidney disease or urinary problems?
- For female patients: How do you cleanse after urination or bowel movements?
- Do you have any physical problems that may affect the urinary tract, such as high blood pressure, diabetes, kidney stones?
- Do you take any vitamins, medications such as antibiotics or diuretics, or eat any particular foods that might cause changes in the characteristics of your urine?
- Do you work in an environment or industry that exposes you to harsh chemicals?

---

[1]From Yoost BL, Crawford LR: *Fundamentals of nursing: Active learning for collaborative practice,* St. Louis, 2016, Mosby.

- Do you experience pain, burning, itching, or other discomfort associated with urination or pain in the sides of your back or abdomen? Describe and rate the pain on a scale of 0 to 10.

HOME CARE RELATED TO URINARY ELIMINATION[2]

- Assess access to toilet facilities. Adequate lighting should be ensured.
- Necessary assistive and safety equipment, such as grab bars and raised toilet seats, should be in place in the home before discharge, as needed. Bedpans and a bedside commode, if warranted, should be in the home ahead of time.
- Supplies necessary for catheterization and catheter care, for urinary diversions, and for incontinence care should be purchased.
- Appropriate referrals to home health or social services should be made before discharge. Services such as home health aides for assistance with activities of daily living (ADLs) should be confirmed.
- Community resources such as the United Ostomy Association and National Association for Continence should be identified as a resource for patients and their families.

[2]From Yoost BL, Crawford LR: *Fundamentals of nursing: Active learning for collaborative practice,* St. Louis, 2016, Mosby.

CHAPTER 37

Death and Loss

STAGES OF DYING AND GRIEF[1]
Denial
- Patient or family may refuse to accept the situation.
- Patient or family may not believe the diagnosis.
- Patient or family may seek second and third opinions.
- Patient or family may claim that the test results were wrong.
- Patient or family may claim that the tests were mixed up with those of someone else.
- Patient may sleep more or be overly talkative or cheerful.

---

[1]From Kübler-Ross E: *On death and dying,* New York, 1969, Collier Books; and Kübler-Ross E: *Questions and answers on death and dying,* New York, 1974, Collier Books.

Anger
- Patient or family may be hostile.
- Patient or family may have excessive demands.
- Patient may be withdrawn, cold, or unemotional.
- Feelings may include envy, resentment, or rage.
- Patient may be angry at family for being well.
- Patient may be uncooperative or manipulative.
- This may be the time that patients are the hardest to care for but the time when they need us the most!

Bargaining
- Patient or family may promise to improve or change habits such as quit smoking, eat less, or exercise more.
- Bargaining may be intertwined with feelings of guilt.
- Bargains are often with the physicians or with God.

Depression
- Patient or family may speak of the upcoming loss.
- Patient or family may cry or weep often.
- Patient or family may want to be alone.

Acceptance
- Patient may exhibit a decreased interest in the surroundings.
- Patient may not want visitors during this time.
- Do not confuse acceptance with depression.
- There seems to be a calmness or peace about the patient.

NURSING INTERVENTIONS RELATED TO DYING AND GRIEF
Denial
This stage is used as a coping or protective function and should not be viewed as a bad quality. It can

be a time when a patient or family can gather their thoughts, feelings, and strengths.

Nursing care:

- Listen, listen, listen (remember, they may talk a lot).
- Get a sense of what they are worried about.
- Be honest with communications.
- Do not give the patient false hope.
- Do not argue with the patient or family.

Anger

This is often directed at caregivers; ensure that caregivers will not stop caring.

Nursing care:

- Do not take anger personally.
- Help family not to take anger personally.
- Visit the patient often and answer call lights promptly.
- Assist the family with much-needed breaks.

Bargaining

Because many of the bargains may be with a divine power, the period may pass unnoticed.

Nursing care:

- Offer frequent chances for the patient or family to talk.
- Offer visits from clergy or other supports.

Depression

Some patients or families may not have a good outlet for their depression.

Nursing care:

- Do not force cheerful or important conversation.
- Allow the patient or family to voice concerns.
- Offer visits from clergy.
- Offer cultural or religious supports.

Acceptance

Patient may want to be alone and families may feel rejected.

Nursing care:

- Encourage family to come often but for brief visits.
- Offer visits from clergy.
- Offer cultural or religious supports.

NURSING INTERVENTIONS RELATED TO IMPENDING DEATH

Personal Care

- Good mouth care: Keep mouth moist; do not use lemon swabs.
- Skin care: Use lotions, massage, good lip care.
- Artificial tears if eyes are open.
- Adequate pain control with medications, massage, and positioning.
- Suction if there are increased secretions to ease breathing.
- Clean and straighten linens often.
- Change position of patient as needed to promote comfort.
- Provide adequate hydration.

Recognize Special Needs

- Encourage visits by clergy.
- Assess for the need for Last Rites, Holy Communion, or other ceremonies.
- Allow for religious music, holy books, and other supports.
- Allow time for the family or friends to pray.
- Encourage cultural or religious rituals or practices.

Prepare the Family

- Describe the physical changes that may be taking place as death approaches.

- Allow the family as much time as possible with the dying patient.
- Offer the family opportunities for cultural or religious rituals.
- Keep the family updated as to the time of approaching death.
- Be honest when telling the family about the impending death.
- Allow for sleep and hygiene needs of the family or friends.
- Allow the family or friends time to voice fears or concerns.
- Allow the family time for questions.
- Allow the family time for tears.

COMMON CULTURAL AND RELIGIOUS DEATH RITUALS[2]

African American
- Friends and family often gather at the home of the deceased to offer support and share in the grief process.
- Wakes with music and singing are common.
- A meal is often shared after the wake and funeral.

Asian American
- Consider practices of the various cultural backgrounds: Chinese, Korean, Japanese, Vietnamese, and Laotian.
- Dying at home may be considered bad luck.
- Respect is shown for the body by providing warm clothes for the burial.
- A shrine to the deceased may be displayed in the home.

---

[2]From End of Life Nursing Education Consortium (ELNEC) Graduate Training Program, 2005, 2011. Retrieved from *www.aacn.nche.edu/ELNEC.*

European American

- Friends and family often gather at the home of the deceased following the death to offer support and share in the grief process.
- Funeral director and clergy assist in planning the funeral and burial.
- Visitation at a funeral home followed by a religious service in a place of worship as well as the gravesite is common.

Hispanic/Latino American

- Diverse cultural backgrounds in this population.
- The rosary is said, often at the home of the deceased.
- Many Hispanic survivors commemorate the loss of a loved one with a promise or commitment that is taken very seriously.

Native American

- Different tribes have different belief systems.
- The Medicine Man or spiritual leader usually moderates the funeral service.
- Some tribes call on their ancestors to come to join the deceased to help with the transition.

Jewish

- Visitors include family, friends, the rabbi, and possibly 10 men from the synagogue; prayers for the sick.
- Body treated with respect. Autopsy discouraged.
- Burial as quickly as possible. Embalming discouraged. Cremation not appropriate.

Islam

- Family and friends visit to provide emotional support.

- After death, body moved to face Mecca if possible.
- Autopsy only for medical or legal reasons.
- Ritualistic washing of the body by a person of the same gender.
- Burial as soon as possible.

Hindu
- Priest, family, and friends visit.
- Grief visually displayed.
- Family may wash the body.
- Cremation preferred, with ashes scattered in sacred rivers.

Buddhist
- Family may bring religious implements: incense, flowers, fruit, prayer beads, or images of Buddha; and may request a teacher or monk.
- Incense is lit in the room.
- Family may wash the body. Cremation is preferred.

Christian
- Family may request a visit from a minister or priest for prayers.
- Sacrament of the Sick may be administered by a Catholic priest.
- Both cremation and burial are acceptable.
- Organ donation and autopsy are permissible.

CARE OF THE BODY AFTER DEATH
If the family is *not* present at the time of death:
- Assess for any special religious, cultural, or family instructions.
- Review the facility's policies and procedure for preparation.

- Assess for any legal limitations in preparing the body.
- Wear gloves when preparing the body.
- The body should be placed flat with the arms and legs straight.
- The eyes and mouth should be closed.
- Remove all intravenous lines, nasogastric tubes, Foley catheters, and so on.
- Clean away any excretions and secretions.
- Dress the body in a clean gown, if possible.
- Remove all excess equipment and trash from room.
- Set personal items (e.g., dentures, glasses) near the patient.
- Pack up all other personal items.
- Document your work in the patient's chart and wait for the family.

If the family is present at the time of death:

- Allow the family time to be with their loved one.
- Ask the family if there are any religious or cultural rituals that need to be honored.
- Ask the family for time to prepare the body.
- Allow the family to assist with the body if they wish.
- Allow the family as much time as possible with the loved one.
- Assist the family in packing up the belongings.
- Assist the family with any paperwork.
- Allow the family to call nonpresent family members, if needed.
- Support the family in deciding on a funeral home or other arrangements.
- After the family has gone, prepare the body for removal per the facility's protocol.
- Document your work in the patient's medical record.

ASSESSMENT OF ANTICIPATORY GRIEF[3]

- Will your loved one's death result in loss of financial support?
- Are you and your family having difficulty making decisions?
- Are there other losses that you are still dealing with?
- Has your loved one's diagnosis or determined prognosis been recent (less than 6 months)?
- Has the illness been of long duration (greater than 12 months)?
- Have you had any suicidal thoughts or do you feel unable to cope with this crisis?

ASSESSMENT OF POTENTIAL DYSFUNCTIONAL GRIEVING[4]

- Do you feel that your support system is inadequate?
- Are you using more alcohol, tobacco, drugs, or prescribed medications?
- Do you have more difficulty sleeping than usual?
- Have you lost or gained weight?
- Has your grief subsided or intensified in the last few weeks?
- Are you able to carry out your day-to-day activities including work, social commitments, and household responsibilities?

[3,4]From Yoost BL, Crawford LR: *Fundamentals of nursing: Active learning for collaborative practice*, St. Louis, 2016, Mosby.

HOME CARE RELATED TO DYING AND GRIEF [5]

Patients receiving hospice in the home require skilled, knowledgeable nurses to provide a high level of quality care as many needs are different for the dying patient and their families. Care includes the following:

- Assessment of safety in the home related to the physical as well as social environment.
- Coordination with all members of the health care team.
- Understanding of any special client request regarding end-of-life wishes.
- Assurances that family care providers are knowledgeable and able to provide the necessary physical care.
- Safe use of equipment that may be used in the home and provision of necessary services.
- Instructions on what to do and who to call at the time of death.
- Prearrangement with funeral home, hospice, clergy, or others who will need to be notified at the time of death.

LEGAL CONSIDERATIONS RELATED TO DEATH

Coroner's case: Deaths in which the county coroner must be made aware, including deaths such as homicides, suicides, and suspicious or accidental deaths.

---

[5]From Yoost BL, Crawford LR: *Fundamentals of nursing: Active learning for collaborative practice*, St. Louis, 2016, Mosby.

Death certificate: The legal document that identifies the date, time, and cause(s) of death.

Documentation: The date and time of death, along with the health care workers' final activities, should be noted in the patient's chart.

Do not resuscitate: Because these words may have different meanings for different people, it should be clearly documented what the meaning is for each patient. Health care facilities should make sure that the wishes of the person and family are being carried out completely and correctly.

Establishing the time of death: Absence of response to external stimuli, heart rate, respiration, and pupillary reflexes.

Final disposition: Final destination for the body. The hospital or county morgue or funeral home is generally the final disposition of the body.

Life-sustaining procedure: Any medical procedure that in the judgment of the physician would only prolong the dying process.

Living Will: A document that informs the physician that in the event of a terminal illness or injury the person wishes to have life-sustaining procedures stopped or withheld.

Organ donations: The law requires all hospitals that receive Medicare dollars to ask for organ donations on death.

Persistent vegetative state: A condition of irreversible cessation of all functions of the cerebral cortex that results in a complete chronic and irreversible cessation of all cognitive functions. This condition must be documented by two physicians.

Postmortem or autopsy: An examination conducted to determine the exact cause of death.

Power of attorney for health care: A legal document in which a person specifies another person to make his or her medical decisions in the event the person cannot.

Pronouncement: Certification as to the time of death. In most states, only a physician is responsible for this procedure.

ORGAN PROCUREMENT
Organs and Tissues That Can Be Donated
Organs
Heart, lungs, liver, pancreas, kidneys, intestines

Bones and Soft Tissues
Humerus, ribs, iliac crest, vertebrae, femur, tibia, fibula, tendons, ligaments, fascia lata

Other Tissues
Eyes, heart valves, skin, saphenous vein

Consent Hierarchy
1. Signed donor card
2. Spouse
3. Adult son or daughter
4. Either parent
5. Adult brother or sister
6. Grandparent
7. Legal guardian

Potential Donors
1. Victims of cerebral trauma
2. Trauma victims
3. Some drug overdose
4. Primary brain tumors

5. Anoxic brain damage
6. Cerebral or subarachnoid bleeds

Special Notes Regarding Procurement

Procuring an organ(s) is a surgical procedure that takes place in the operating room under sterile conditions.

When applicable, after the procurement, prosthetic replacement and proper suturing are completed to restore the body to its natural appearance. Donating organs should not interfere with funeral arrangements or with the desire to have an open-casket funeral. There is no cost to the donating family for the procurement or transplant procedure.

CULTURAL AND RELIGIOUS CONSIDERATIONS AFTER DEATH

	Accepts Autopsies	Burial vs. Cremation	May Donate Organs
Agnostic	Yes	Both	Yes
Amish	Yes	Burial	Reluctant
Arab	Discouraged	Burial	Reluctant
Atheist	Yes	Both	Yes
Baha'i	Yes	Burial	Yes
Buddhist	Yes	Cremation	Yes
Cambodian	Yes	Both	Yes
Catholic (Orthodox)	Reluctant	Burial	Reluctant
Catholic (Roman)	Yes	Both	Yes
Chinese	Yes	Both	Yes
Christian	Yes	Both	Yes

Christian Scientist	Reluctant	Both	Reluctant
Eastern Orthodox	Reluctant	Burial	Yes
Filipino	Yes	Both	Yes
Gypsy	Reluctant	Burial	Reluctant
Hindu	Reluctant	Both	Yes
Hispanic	Yes	Both	Yes
Hmong	Yes	Both	Yes
Islamic	Reluctant	Burial	Reluctant
Japanese	Yes	Both	Yes
Jehovah's Witness	Reluctant	Both	Reluctant
Judaism (Hasidim)	Reluctant	Burial	Reluctant
Judaism (Orthodox)	Reluctant	Burial	Reluctant
Judaism (Reform)	Yes	Both	Yes
Korean	Yes	Both	Reluctant
Laotian	Yes	Both	Yes
Mennonite	Yes	Both	Yes

Continued

00 8

052400000ни00

CULTURAL AND RELIGIOUS CONSIDERATIONS AFTER DEATH—cont'd

	Accepts Autopsies	Burial vs. Cremation	May Donate Organs
Mormon	Yes	Burial	Yes
Native American	Reluctant	Both	Reluctant
Quaker	Yes	Cremation	Yes
Russian Orthodox	Yes	Both	Yes
Seventh Day Adventist	Reluctant	Both	Yes
Shinto	No	Both	No
Sikhism	Reluctant	Stillborn: Burial All others: Cremated	Yes
Taoist	Yes	Both	Yes
Thai	Yes	Both	Yes
Vietnamese	Yes	Cremation	Yes

Index

Note: Page numbers followed by *f* indicate figures and *t* indicate tables respectively.

Fiber, benefits of, 275
Fibrinogen split products (FSP),
    reference range of, 225*t*
Filipino, cultural and religious
    considerations of, after
    death, 308*t*
Final disposition, after death, 305
Finger abduction, as range of
    motion, 183
Finger adduction, as range of
    motion, 183
Finger extension, as range of
    motion, 183
Finger flexion, as range of motion,
    183
Fingertips, for palpation, 46
Fire safety, 142
Fistulas, wound healing and, 195
Five rights of delegation, 83–84
Five wishes, 80
Flow sheets, 63
Fluid(s), 261–270
    of body, 67
    volume
        average intake and output of,
            263, 263*t*
        deficit of, 261–262
        excess of, 262
Fluoroscopy, 223
Focus, on one problem/issue, as
    nursing diagnostic process, 49
Focused questions, 39
Folic acid (folate), 240. *see also*
    Vitamin B$_9$
Foot, problems of, 191–192
Forced expiratory flow (FEF), 253
Forced expiratory volume in one
    second (FEV$_1$), 253
Forced vital capacity (FVC), 253
Form, definition of, 233
Formal operations, 91*t*
Formats, of documentation, 62–63
Forms, of documentation, 63
Fowler, patient positioning, 186
FRC. *see* Functional residual
    capacity (FRC).
Frequency
    as fecal characteristics, 272*t*
    of voice, 22

Friction rub, 252
    pericardial, 109–110
    pleural, 112
Frostbite, 104
Full liquid diet, 199*t*
Function urinary incontinence, 287*t*
Functional assessment, 41–43
Functional residual capacity (FRC),
    254
Fungal infection(s)
    fever in, 103
    of foot, 191–192
Fungi, definition of, 158
FVC. *see* Forced vital capacity
    (FVC).

G

Gastrectomy, 242
Gastrointestinal system,
    assessment of, 46, 249
Gastroplasty, 242
Gay, 136
Gender
    plan of care and, 51–52
    pulse rate and, 106
    roles, definition of, 136
Generalized tonic-clonic seizure,
    144
Genetic difference, definition of, 233
Genital herpes, 138
Genitourinary system, assessment
    of, 46, 248
German measles, 168
Gestures, for effective
    communication, 21
GI series, 223
Glass thermometer, reading, 102
Glaucoma, 209
Glossopharyngeal nerve, 120–122
Glucose
    range of, 226*t*
    testing
        home care considerations
            for, 232
        in urinary elimination, 291
Glucose tolerance, in timed urine
    tests, 292
Glucose tolerance test (GTT), 223